HOW TO PREVENT BREAST CANCER

BEFORE & AFTER

A GUIDE TO TAKING BACK CONTROL OF YOUR LIFE

Pamela Wartian Smith, MD, MPH

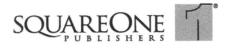
SQUAREONE
PUBLISHERS

Editor: Erica Shur
Typesetting: Gary A. Rosenberg

The information and advice contained in this book are based upon the research and the personal and professional experiences of the author. They are not intended as a substitute for consulting with a healthcare professional. The publisher and author are not responsible for any adverse effects or consequences resulting from the use of any of the suggestions, preparations, or procedures discussed in this book. All matters pertaining to your physical health should be supervised by a healthcare professional. It is a sign of wisdom, not cowardice, to seek a second or third opinion.

Square One Publishers
115 Herricks Road Garden City Park, NY 11040
(516) 535-2010 (877) 900-BOOK
www.squareonepublishers.com

Library of Congress Cataloging-in-Publication Data
Name: Smith, Pamela Wartian, author.
Title: How to prevent breast cancer before and after / Pamela
    W. Smith, MD, MPH, MS.
Description: Garden City Park, NY: Square One Publishers, [2025] |
Includes bibliographical references and index. | Summary: "In Part 1
    of the book, you will learn about the four different types of breast
    cancer. The controllable risk factors to prevent and stop a reocurrence
    of breast cancer are outlined along with the uncontrollable risk factors,
    such as heredity, age, environment, and lifestyle. The last section deals
    with immunity and how your immune system works."— Provided by publisher.
Identifiers: LCCN 2024027867 | ISBN 9780757005350 (paperback) | ISBN
    9780757055355 (epub)
Subjects: LCSH: Breast—Cancer—Prevention—Popular works. |
    Breast—Cancer—Relapse—Popular works. | Breast—Cancer—Popular works.
Classification: LCC RC280.B8 S65 2024 | DDC 616.99/449—dc23/eng/20241112
LC record available at https://lccn.loc.gov/2024027867

Printed in the United States of America

10   9   8   7   6   5   4   3   2   1

This book is dedicated to Rebecca Duchene,
who fought the good fight against breast cancer
and has now gone on to be with the Lord in Heaven.

She was one of the most gracious and kind people
in the world. Everyone who knew her saw
the Lord shining through her.

May she rest in peace.

Contents

Acknowledgments

To Michael Holick, PhD, MD, an endocrinologist whose pioneering work in vitamin D led to the identification of both calcidiol, the major circulating form of vitamin D, and calcitriol, the active form of vitamin D.

To David Zava, PhD, a biochemist and researcher whose groundbreaking work on hormones and breast cancer has changed the face of medicine.

To Rudy Shur, who took a chance many years ago on this struggling author. Medicine and the world are a better place for all the fabulous books he has published over the years.

To Erica Shur, an editor who has helped me grow as a writer and helped me embrace the ability to write for both the public and health care providers in the same manuscript.

Writing a book is harder than I thought, and more rewarding than I could have ever imagined, when I wrote my first book twenty years ago. None of this would have been possible without my best friend and lover, my husband Christopher. He stood by me during every struggle and all my successes. He is a true partner in life. I am so very blessed.

Preface

Writing this book has been a labor of love. I personally have a history of breast cancer on both sides of my family. On my father's side, I never met my grandmother. She died of breast cancer before I was born. I also had a cousin on the same side of the family that passed away from the disease. On my mother's side of my family, I had two aunts with this disease process. One died of breast cancer, and the other beat the cancer. I also have a cousin on that side of the family who is currently being treated for breast cancer, as is my best friend.

I have the great fortune to have the world's best editor, Erica Shur, and the world's best publisher, Rudy Shur. They have helped me through this book in ways that no other editor or publisher could. This book could not have been written without their enormous help.

It is my hope, in writing this book, that all women not only learn more about their own bodies but that you, the reader, learn that there are risk factors for breast cancer that are unchangeable. Fortunately, there are also many more risk factors that you can control, you can modify, you can improve, and even totally change.

This book was written to empower women of all ages—to help women significantly lower their risk of developing breast cancer, and if you have already had this disease, to decrease your risk of its reoccurrence. Take control of your own health; science is here to help you. Remember, to be truly healthy, you must be physically healthy, emotionally healthy, and spiritually healthy.

Pamela W. Smith, MD, MPH, MS

PART 1

What to Know About Breast Cancer

1

Breast Cancer Basics

Breast cancer is the most common cancer diagnosed in women, account-ing for more than 1 in 10 new cancer diagnoses each year. Breast cancer commonly develops silently, and most of the time it's discovered during routine screenings. While your doctor will play an important role in its detec-tion and treatment, it is also important to understand what is going on, and what your options are as a patient. In Part 1 of this book, we will examine the signs and symptoms of breast cancer, the various types of breast cancer, the changes that occur in the cells as well as how the disease is evaluated and diagnosed (including the newest methods therein). We will also look at the conventional therapies used to treat breast cancer. First, however, let's under-stand what cancer is.

WHAT IS CANCER?

Our bodies are made up of millions of cells. All these cells have specific pur-poses. When one cell dies, another cell reproduces to replace the old cell. As we get older, the process tends to slow down. This accounts for gray hair, wrinkles, and lots of other things we associate with aging. The problem occurs when the cells begin to reproduce in an uncontrollable manner. This can happen in any part of our body—in any of our organs, in our blood, on our skin—and in the breast. This is what cancer is. As we will see in Part 2, this happens for many reasons. Some risk factors are difficult to control, while others are not.

The mechanics of this can be explained in a simple way. All cells have sensing "antennas" called *receptors* that are composed of protein molecules. These receptors receive signaling instructions from other molecules that attach to these receptors. These other molecules circulate throughout the body and can come from many different sources such as hormones, nutrients, drugs, viruses, and more. The signals they send follow a *pathway*, which is made up of a series of chemical interactions that provide any number of messages to the cell. It is the message of these signals that determine the internal behavior of a cell.

These signals can provide instructions for the cell to continue its normal daily activities. Or signals can be harmful, instructing the cell to multiply in place, growing into a benign or cancerous mass or tumor. These types of tumors are called *in situ*—Latin for "in place." While there may be more than one mass, they seem to be localized, referred to as *non-invasive*. They can certainly do damage, but they tend not to spread to other parts of the body. However, some cancers are aggressive. While they are formed in one part of the body, they can spread to other parts. The process is called *metastasis*. Some of these types of cancers can move slowly, while other forms can be very aggressive.

On the other hand, a cell may have a pre-existing trigger that, when set off in any number of ways, develops into cancer. This may be at the root cause of inherited cancer cells. Whatever way a growth may be formed, it's important to remember that by doing monthly breast self-examinations, you can potentially detect it in its early stages. This should not replace regular mammograms and/or medical exams.

SELF-EXAMINATIONS

Every woman should know the signs and symptoms of breast cancer. Starting in your late teens or early twenties, performing monthly self-examinations will help to more easily identify any changes in your breasts. Knowing how your breasts normally look and feel will help you identify any changes or abnormalities. Be sure to talk to your healthcare provider if you notice anything unusual.

SIGNS AND SYMPTOMS OF BREAST CANCER

The most common symptom of breast cancer is a new lump or thickened area of skin that feels different from the area around it. Remember that most lumps or masses are not cancerous. A painless, hard mass that has irregular edges is more likely to be cancer. However, breast cancer lumps can be round, tender, softer, and/or painful. But they all need to be evaluated. Other symptoms, according to the American Cancer Society, include the following:

☐ Breast or nipple pain

☐ Nipple discharge (other than breast milk)

☐ Nipple or breast skin that is red, dry, flaking, or thickened

☐ Nipple retraction (turning inward)

☐ Skin dimpling (sometimes looking like an orange peel)

☐ Swelling of all or part of a breast (even if no lump is felt)

☐ Swollen lymph nodes under the arm or near the collarbone (sometimes this can be a sign of breast cancer spreading even before the original tumor in the breast is large enough to be felt)

ANATOMY OF A WOMAN'S BREAST

Women's breasts are composed of several types of tissues. They include:

- **Adipose tissue**. This is the fatty tissue that makes up the majority of the breast.

- **Areolae**. This is the darker-colored circular area surrounding the nipple.

- **Blood vessels**. Circulates blood throughout the breasts.

- **Connective or fibrous tissue**. This tissue acts to provide support to the breast.

- **Glandular tissue**. Inside the lobes are small glands that produce milk.

- **Lobes**. These are the small milk-producing sacs that surround the nipple.

- **Lymph nodes**. These glands function as filters, help fight infections, and act as markers to indicate the stage of a cancer.

- **Lymph vessels**. Circulates the lymphatic fluid running throughout the body.

- **Milk ducts**. These are the small tubes that carry milk from the lobes to the nipples.

- **Montgomery glands**. Found inside the areolae, these glands create a lubricant oil that protects the nipple from chafing during breastfeeding.

- **Nerves**. Provides sensitivity to the surrounding skin and nipples of the breast.

While any of the tissues listed above can become cancerous, the cells lining the milk ducts, along with the lobes, are the most commonly affected. It is also important to point out that a number of these breast cells may be subject to producing non-cancerous (benign) symptoms such as breast lumps, pain, and nipple discharge. Let's consider some of these common conditions.

BENIGN BREAST CONDITIONS

Benign breast conditions may appear in several different ways. These conditions include breast pain, palpable masses, nipple discharge, and inflammatory lesions. Breast pain is one of the most common symptoms. Many women will experience it at some point. Most of the pain is self-limited and resolves quickly. If it persists for more than a week, make sure you see your primary care physician or other healthcare provider.

EARLY WARNING SIGNS

There are several benign breast conditions to be considered. Signs and symptoms of these conditions range from pain and abnormal physical examination findings to asymptomatic abnormalities detected in breast imaging studies. Many benign breast conditions are diagnosed and managed by primary care physicians, but some patients may require consultation with a breast subspecialist.

- **Inflammatory breast lesions** may be benign, infectious in nature, or a sign of malignancy. They should be evaluated by your doctor right away.

- **Nipple discharge** is a common occurrence. It accounts for two to five percent of medical visits by women. In fact, as many as 80 percent of women will experience at least one episode of nipple discharge during their lifetime. It is the presenting symptom of 5 to 12 percent of breast cancers and therefore if you have this symptom, make sure that you see your primary care physician as soon as possible. Your primary care healthcare provider will work with radiologists and surgeons to assess and treat the nipple discharge.

- **Palpable masses** may be found by yourself or on routine physical examination. Your healthcare provider will want to know how long the mass has been there and if it has changed in size over time. It may be associated with pain, and it may change in size with different times in your menstrual cycle. Any masses should be evaluated by your healthcare provider as soon as possible.

The bottom line is to have these symptoms checked out by a physician. In most instances, many of the tools used to determine if the tissue is benign are the same tools used to see if the tissue is cancerous.

DIAGNOSIS OF BREAST CANCER

Breast cancer diagnosis often begins with your healthcare provider examining your breasts and discussing your symptoms. However, many women with breast cancer have no symptoms. Therefore, regular breast cancer is critical. The key to successful treatment of breast cancer is early diagnosis.

DIAGNOSTIC TOOLS

There are different imaging machines and tests to aid in the diagnosis of breast cancer. These include X-ray, ultrasound, magnetic resonance imaging (MRI), and nuclear medicine.

▉ X-Ray: Mammogram

A mammogram is an x-ray of the breast that can reveal *benign* (non-cancerous) or *malignant* (cancerous) abnormalities. Mammograms can be utilized for both screening and diagnosis. Mammogram screening is performed as an attempt to detect any early signs of breast cancer, even before symptoms occur. It is also commonly used to detect breast cancer if a woman experiences symptoms, such as a lump that can be felt in the breast. And yet, while mammography screenings have proven to be effective, the potential drawbacks of this technique have also been commonly discussed in medicine, since it relies on subjective human interpretation. They include:

- False-positive recalls leading to additional imaging studies or biopsies that can increase the expense, exposure to radiation, and cause the patient a great deal of stress.

- False-negatives when breast cancers are either not seen on mammography because of dense breasts or there was an error made by the radiologist on interpretation.

What Is a Dense Breast?

Breasts are composed of milk glands, milk ducts, supportive tissue, fibrous tissue, and fat cells. The more of these cells you have within a given space, the denser the breast tissue. A mammogram image provides an accurate picture of how dense a breast is. Tissue density ranges from normal to extreme density. (See Chapter 3, "Unchangeable Risk Factors for Breast Cancer," page 55 for more information.)

There are, however, two new methods of using mammograms to help pinpoint growths in the breasts. They are the use of Artificial Intelligence (AI) and Contrast-Enhanced Mammograms (CEM).

Artificial Intelligence (AI). Artificial intelligence (AI) is currently being used in several aspects of radiology, including interpretation of mammograms. The medical literature is mixed on the efficacy of AI for this purpose. Some articles reveal that the use of AI increases cancer detection and reduces false positives, thus its increasing. However, other studies suggest that AI and its use in mammography is not yet ready for prime time since the technique is only as good as the people that are programming it. Perhaps the best of both worlds is needed where there is a combination of artificial intelligence and radiologist reading.

Contrast-Enhanced Mammograms (CEM). Contrast-enhanced mammograms are used when traditional mammograms are done with IV contrast material that is *iodinated*—in other words, it contains iodine. This technique is used in place of an MRI of the breast without the additional expense and IV gadolinium that is used with MRIs. Iodine is considered a less toxic form of contrast than using gadolinium. CEM is also a better technique for individuals who are claustrophobic.

This technique may be used to determine the extent of the disease in a person recently diagnosed with breast cancer. It may also be used to monitor the response to a treatment or to evaluate the breast after treatment for residual or recurrent disease. In addition, CEM can detect abnormal structural changes as well as new vascular changes that are commonly associated with breast cancer. Furthermore, contrast-enhanced mammograms may be used as a potential screening in women who are at intermediate- or high-risk for breast cancer.

■ Thermography

Despite some limitations, mammography is the gold standard for screening breast malignancy. Another emerging method for screening is *thermography*. Digital infrared thermal imaging is the thermography used to also diagnose breast cancer. The concept behind this test is that as cancer cells multiply, they need more oxygen-rich blood for growth. As there is an increase in blood flow to the tumor, the temperature around the tumor also increases. Malignant cells discharge nitric oxide into the bloodstream and cause impairment in the circulation of the blood in the smallest blood vessels. The released nitric oxide, along with the active growth of cancerous cells, increase blood circulation and temperature in that region.

Evaluating these differences in temperature leads to the detection of the malignant area in the breast. In other words, thermography captures heat map images of the target surface through an infrared camera, which helps to detect malignancy. With recent developments in thermal sensors, imaging protocols, and computer-aided software, there is now promise for making this technique a mainstream screening method for cancer.

Ultrasound

Breast ultrasound is an imaging test that uses sound waves to look at the inside of your breasts. Although mammography is a gold standard for breast cancer imaging, because of its limitations regarding dense breasts, another supplementing screening tool is required. Ultrasound is a supplemental tool that may be utilized to analyze some breast changes in women with dense breast tissues, as well as suspicious areas not seen on a mammogram. Advantages of this technique include its wide availability, as well as no patient exposure to radiation.

At the same time, however, it is limited by several factors. Most notably, it may fail to detect *microcalcifications* (a tiny deposit of calcium in the breast), and it may miss some early signs of cancer. Because of these limitations, this technique is not used to screen for breast cancer and is reserved for special situations. The fusion of ultrasound with other modalities, such as ultrasound imaging techniques and ultrasound-guided biopsy, provide important tools for the management of breast cancer patients.

Ultrasound elastography is now a routine noninvasive tool used to measure the consistency or hardness of the tissues to differentiate benign and malignant breast lesions. Contrast-enhanced ultrasound and other modalities fused with ultrasound are other tools that may be useful in the noninvasive prediction of prognostic factors of breast cancer. Complementary high-resolution ultrasound is excellent for detecting breast lesions when in expert hands. Based on existing literature, it was found that fusion of other modalities with ultrasound may be an effective primary detection tool for breast lesions, particularly in low- and middle-income countries with low-resource settings and where mammography and other expensive techniques are not available.

Magnetic Resonance Imaging (MRI)

Magnetic resonance imaging (MRIs) are diagnostic tests using magnetic fields (as those produced by magnets) and radio waves to create internal images of the breast. These machines are more sensitive in detecting possible cancer growths than mammograms. They include:

Diffusion-Weighted Imaging (DWI). Diffusion-weighted imaging is a form of unenhanced MRI that uses the diffusion of water molecules to generate contrast in MRI images to address some of the shortcomings faced by a regular breast MRI. The potential benefits of DWI techniques include improved differentiation of benign and malignant breast lesions and assessment and prediction of therapeutic efficacy. Technical innovations are helping to overcome many of the image-quality issues that have limited widespread use of DWI for the breast. While DWI may be an accurate and nonradioactive imaging technique, it has still not achieved its full potential.

Dynamic Contrast-Enhanced MRI (DCE-MRI). Dynamic contrast-enhanced breast MRI works by analyzing the temporal enhancement pattern (an increase in signal intensity) of a tissue following the intravenous injection of a paramagnetic contrast agent. This non-invasive imaging technique quantitatively determines the extent of tissue vascularization, interstitial space composition (space that lies between blood vessels and cells, thereby providing the fluid that surrounds the cells), and differentiation of lesions. This imaging modality is useful to depict tumor angiogenesis with overall reoccurrence and overall survival of breast cancer patients.

DCE-MRI technique is non-invasive and three-dimensional, which allows visualization of the extent of disease before morphological alterations. This helps to predict the overall response either before the start of therapy or early during treatment. Unlike mammography, DCE-MRI is not limited by breast tissue density. However, a major limitation of DCE-MRI is that it is non-specific.

Magnetic Resonance Elastography (MRE). Magnetic resonance elastography can be used to obtain details on tissue mechanical properties *in vivo* (inside the living body). Following application of an external stress, breast MRE, a non-invasive, non-ionizing, and cross-sectional imaging modality, can quantitate the *viscoelastic* (material that behaves like both a liquid and solid) properties of breast tissues.

Breast cancers often have a higher stiffness due to an increase in the number of cells, collagen, and *proteoglycans* (proteins) compared to the normal surrounding tissues and benign lesions. While the initial results are encouraging, the most significant limitation for MRE in breast cancer is spatial resolution and detection of small focal lesions due to the overlap in the soft malignant tumors and stiff benign lesions' elasticity ranges.

Magnetic Resonance Imaging (MRI). Breast MRI is a non-invasive and non-ionizing diagnostic imaging tool that employs low-energy radio frequency waves and a magnetic field to obtain detailed images of structures within the breast. MRI can be used to measure the size of the cancer and look for metastasized tumors in women who have been previously diagnosed with breast cancer. Tumors with a size less than or equal to 2 centimeters (cm) have been accurately identified and measured using MRI.

Magnetic Resonance Spectroscopy (MRS). Magnetic resonance spectroscopy can measure a chemical "spectrum" in the region using high magnetic field strengths (typically 11–14 T) on body fluids, cell extracts, and tissue samples, providing additional information about the chemical content in the region. There has been considerable progress on breast MRS in the last decade; however, multiple factors can potentially limit MRS.

Nuclear Medicine Studies

These types of imaging machines use radioactive material and specialized cameras to take pictures of the breast. This is done because cancer cells attract more radioactive material than healthy breast cells. There are several types of these machines. They include:

Breast Specific Gamma Imaging (BSGI). Breast specific gamma imaging, a molecular breast imaging approach, is a specialized nuclear medicine imaging test that allows detection of sub-centimeter and mammographically occult (found in one or more metastatic sites but the primary site is hidden) breast cancer with a sensitivity and specificity comparable to MRI. In BSGI, a radiotracer, such as Technetium Tc99m Sestamibi, is injected into the patient's bloodstream and the breast is visualized using a special camera. Unlike mammography, BSGI is unaffected by breast density. The major drawback of this technique is that since the entire body gets exposed to the radiation, it is not possible to use this method of testing frequently.

Molecular Image-Guided Sentinel Lymph Node Biopsy (SLNB). Sentinel lymph node biopsy is a revolutionary, minimally-invasive method to determine whether metastasis has occurred in early-stage breast cancer patients. SLNB technique is well known for its significantly reduced post-operative complications associated with conventional axillary lymph node dissection.

Positron Emission Tomography (PET) Scanning and PET in Conjunction with Computer-aided Tomography (CT) Scanning (PET-CT). Positron emission tomography imaging, commonly called a PET scan, has been widely adopted as an important clinical modality for oncology. PET radiotracers take advantage of the enhanced glucose metabolism of cancer cells. Cancerous cells are highly proliferative and have a higher glucose metabolism rate than normal cells. FDG (fluorodeoxyglucose) PET radiotracers enter cells through the glucose transporter and are, thus, taken up in greater amounts by tumor cells than by healthy cells. FDG uptake inversely correlates with prognosis.

PET-CT is a combination of PET (a nuclear medicine technique) and CT that produces highly detailed views of the body. The improved spatial resolution and sensitivity of PET scanners dedicated to the breast (positron emission mammography) has allowed its clinical application in the study of primary tumors. Physicians use PET-CT studies to diagnose and stage cancer, plan your treatment, evaluate the effectiveness of treatment, and manage ongoing care.

Theranostic Imaging. One of the intensively developing fields is nuclear medicine, combining molecular diagnostic imaging and subsequent (radio)therapy in the light of theranostics. *Theranostics* has emerged as a new paradigm for the simultaneous diagnosis, imaging, and treatment of cancers. It has the potential to provide timely and improved patient care through personalized therapy. In nanotheranostics, cell-specific targeting *moieties* (a major half of a molecule), imaging agents, and therapeutic agents can be embedded within a single formulation for effective treatment.

■ Ki-67 TESTING

The *Ki-67 test* is designed to help measure how fast the cancer cells are growing and dividing. It is one of the latest tests available. Ki-67 is a protein found in the nucleus of cancer cells that are actively growing and dividing. Recently, in evaluating breast cancer, Ki-67 is one of the main tumor markers that your healthcare provider will check for when diagnosing, staging, and monitoring the cancer. A higher level of Ki-67 means that the cancer cells are multiplying at a faster rate. Thus, knowing how much Ki-67 is produced by your tumor can help your healthcare team estimate how likely the cancer is to grow and spread.

Use of the Ki-67 test in breast cancer remains controversial, but it is becoming more commonly ordered by oncologists. This test uses an antibody that attaches to antigen receptors on the Ki-67 protein. The higher the concentration of Ki-67, the more the cells will absorb the antibody material and be visible under the microscope on tissue obtained from a biopsy.

Research is underway to determine how to best apply the information from the test to patient care. Some studies have found that tumors with higher levels of Ki-67 may have a worse prognosis than tumors with lower levels. Positively, studies have found that tumors with a high level of Ki-67 may respond particularly well to chemotherapy. In test results, you will see the Ki-67 findings expressed as a percentage. This is the percentage of the total sample that has active Ki-67 proteins. This is used to estimate how many cells are actively dividing. Less than five percent is considered low. Thirty percent

(30%) or higher is considered high. While healthcare providers increasingly order the Ki-67 proliferation marker test, its overall benefit is still uncertain.

EVALUATING BREAST CANCERS

Once breast cancer has been diagnosed, there are a number of factors to consider. A number of tests can be given to determine how advanced the cancer is and to identify the specific type of breast cancer cell. These tests include the following:

- **Tumor size.** When imaging a breast cancer tumor, the tumor is measured at its wide point in millimeters (*mm*) or centimeters (*cm*) to determine its size. This measurement is used to determine its stage and to decide on the treatment options.

- **Grade.** A pathologist examines the tumor under a microscope and grades it from 1 to 3 in comparison to a normal cell. The greater the number, the more likely it is to spread. For example, a small localized tumor that has not spread is referred as a T1. These tumors measuring less than 2 cm in diameter have a ten-year survival rate of approximately 85 percent. A tumor that is larger than 5 centimeters is referred to as a T3 tumor. In some instances, it is the result of a delayed diagnosis, and statically, has a ten-year survival rate of less than 60 percent. T4 indicates that the tumor has metastasized and has spread.

- **Regional lymph node infiltration.** This is done when a doctor feels for enlarged lymph nodes under the arm, through imaging to detect enlarged nodes, and through a needle biopsy.

- **Histology.** The process uses a biopsy to identify breast cancer cells through microscopic examination.

- **Immunohistochemistry (IHC).** The body's immune system produces proteins, called *antibodies*, to fight off harmful microscopic substances called *antigens*. Specific antigens are found on the surface of a cancerous cell. This laboratory test uses antibodies to identify cancerous antigens or markers taken from a tissue sample. Based on the findings, it can provide characteristics of the cancer type to determine the best options for treatment.

- **Evaluation of estrogen receptor (ER).** Found on the outside of a cell, a cell receptor is a protein molecule that receives and responds to signals from inside and outside a cell. In a normal breast cell, the cell produces these receptors in order for the cell to function normally. When a receptor on a cancerous cell binds to a specific hormone, it can stimulate the cancer to grow. This test detects whether the breast cancer cells have receptors that attach the hormone estrogen, which allows the cancer to grow and multiply.

- **Evaluation of progesterone receptor (PR).** This test determines whether breast cancer cells have receptors that attach to the hormone progesterone, which allows the cancer to grow and reproduce.

- **Human epidermal growth factor receptor 2 (HER2).** The human epidermal growth factor receptor (EGFR) is a protein receptor that regulates division and survival in normal cells. As a receptor, it binds with other molecules and atoms to determine a cell's behavior. In breast cancer cells, the HER2 is a protein that increases cell growth. In cells with high levels of these proteins, called *HER2 positive*, cancer cells grow more rapidly and spread quickly. In *HER2 negative* cells, there are no abnormal levels of this protein, and the growth is slower. This test measures the level of HER2 to see whether the cell is HER2 positive or negative.

- **Proliferation marker Ki-67.** This is another protein that indicates the rate of cell division in a tumor. It is a marker to help indicate how the breast cancer will respond to specific treatments.

These factors are the most significant prognostic and therapeutic predictors in current breast cancer clinical practice.

TYPES OF BREAST CANCERS

For many years, breast cancer has been divided into two categories. The first is *non-invasive* and the second is *invasive*. Non-invasive indicates that the cancer will stay in place and not spread, while invasive will spread.

NON-INVASIVE

Ductal Carcinoma in Situ (DCIS)

Ductal carcinoma in situ (DCIS) is a non-invasive early stage of breast cancer.

It is most commonly a non-invasive cancer cell. These cells develop in the lining of the breast milk ducts. They have a low risk of spreading. It is usually found during a mammogram or detected as a breast lump. There are usually no other symptoms. When found, it is graded as a stage 0 breast cancer. About 1 in 5 new breast cancers will be DCIS. With that said, some forms of DCIS can become invasive, so it is important to find an appropriate treatment.

INVASIVE

▣ Invasive Ductal Carcinoma (IDC)

Invasive ductal carcinoma (IDC) is the most common form of breast cancer, accounting for about 70 to 80 percent of all cases. It forms in the milk ducts and grows into other parts of the breast. It can also spread to other parts of the body. Symptoms may appear as a lump or thickening in the breast or it may cause redness, scales, dimpling, or a rash around the nipple or breast. Nipples may turn inward or produce a non-milk discharge. There may also be a lump or swelling in the underarm. It can be detected by mammogram and biopsy.

▣ Invasive Lobular Carcinoma (ILC)

This is the second most common form of breast cancer, accounting for approximately 5 to 10 percent of all cases. It begins in the lobules and may then spread to surrounding tissues as well as other parts of the body. ILC causes a thickening or hardening of the connective tissue in the breast. It can also produce color changes on the breast skin and nipple. It is not easily detected on a mammogram. A needle biopsy test is commonly used to identify ILC.

▣ Inflammatory Breast Cancer (IBC)

This cancer makes up about 1 to 5 percent of breast cancers, which can be detected in the ducts or lobules of a breast. As these cancer cells grow, they block the lymph vessels in the skin of the breast and cause inflammation. Symptoms may show as redness and dimpling on the surface of the breast. It may also produce a rapid increase in breast size, tenderness in the breast, or an inverted nipple. It may also not show up on a mammogram. Biopsy and other forms of imaging may be needed to confirm a diagnosis.

IMMUNOHISTOCHEMICAL (IHC) CLASSIFICATIONS OF BREAST CANCERS

With the advancements in genetic analysis, there is a new way to classify breast cancers based on their protein receptors. These are the "antennas" that these various molecules look for. This system overlaps the classifications mentioned above. It is based on the genetic makeup of the breast cancer cell and is now used to determine more effective treatments. There are four major IHC classifications of breast cancers, based on whether they have hormone receptors identifying them as positive or whether they lack these receptors describing them as negative. These include:

- **Endocrine receptor** (estrogen or progesterone receptor) positive (BRER)

- **Human epidermal growth factor receptor 2 positive**, commonly called HER2 positive (BRHR)

- **Triple positive** composed of estrogen, progesterone, and HER2 positive receptors (BRTP)

- **Triple negative**, which has an absence of estrogen, progesterone, and HER2 receptors (BRTN)

These four types have specific outcomes (prognoses) and responses to therapy. For example, the hormone receptor positive breast cancers (BRER, BRTP) respond to endocrine therapy and show better prognoses, while the hormone receptor negative types (BRHR, BRTN) are more aggressive, non-responsive to endocrine therapy and have poorer prognoses.

When Breast Cancer Spreads

Metastasis is the process by which breast cancer cells may have spread from its original site in the breast to other parts of the body. The signs and symptoms of this spread will depend on where the cancer has spread. The most common areas breast cancer may spread to are bone, brain, liver, and lung, although breast cancer can spread to almost any part of the body.

1. **Bone metastases** produce progressive aching and pain in the area of bone where the cancer has spread. Sometimes individuals are not aware of spread to the bone until they fracture it.

2. **Liver metastases** are commonly suspected when the person's liver enzymes on their blood tests have started to elevate, and the patient commonly starts itching. They may also experience *jaundice* (yellow discoloration of the skin and the whites of the eyes). Nausea, vomiting, and stomach pain may also occur.

3. **Lung metastases** from breast cancer may cause a chronic cough and shortness of breath that becomes progressive. A buildup of fluid between the membranes lining the lung may also occur. This is called a *pleural effusion*.

4. **Brain metastases** is when the cancer spreads to the brain. Headaches, dizziness, visual changes, seizures, and even personality changes may occur.

CONVENTIONAL TREATMENTS FOR BREAST CANCER

Medical research for breast cancer diagnosis and treatments started in the nineteenth century. Today, with a greater understanding of genetics and the use of Artificial Intelligence, diagnostic methods have greatly improved along with the number of treatments.

Surgery

Breast cancer surgery refers to the removal of the entire breast, called a *mastectomy*, or some part of the breast in a procedure called a *lumpectomy*. The amount of the breast removed is based upon the size of the tumor, its location, and the type of cancer found. Sometimes lymph nodes may also be removed to see if the cancer has spread. In a radical mastectomy, the entire breast is removed while all the lymph nodes under the arm are taken out along with the chest wall muscles under the breast. This procedure may be followed up by radiation treatments and/or drug therapies.

Cryoablation

One of the newest conventional treatments for breast cancer is the use of extreme cold to destroy abnormal cells. The procedure is called *cryoablation*. It is also called percutaneous cryoablation, cryosurgery, or cryotherapy. This method of removal has the advantage of being a minimally invasive procedure useful in early breast cancer and metastatic breast cancer when surgery is not an option. Cryoablation consists of cycles of first freeze, a thaw phase, and a second freeze. It usually takes less than 45 minutes to be completed. Breast cryoablation may be done with ultrasound, CT scan, or MRI guidance. Cryoablation can be carried out with little anesthesia because the cooling produced by the probes provides analgesia. In addition, it does not interrupt other systemic therapies.

Possible side effects of this mode of treatment can occur, such as fat necrosis and infection. Fat necrosis is a noncancerous lump in the breast that develops from dead or damaged breast tissue. Skin necrosis (tissue death that occurs when blood flow to your body tissues is blocked) or pectoralis muscle necrosis has been reported rarely. Other minor adverse effects include breast pain, swelling, ecchymosis (discoloration of the skin), and skin burns.

Most studies suggest that due to the small sample size of the current research, reliable conclusions cannot be drawn on this mode of treatment and more research needs to be completed.

■ Radiation Therapy (Radiotherapy)

After surgery, to reduce the reoccurrence of cancer, radiation therapy is given to the patient. In this treatment, high energy radioactive beams are projected on the area having been exposed to the cancer cells. The standard schedule of treatment is usually five days a week, for six to seven weeks. Side effects from this treatment may include breast pain and swelling, redness, peeling skin, infection, fatigue, a collection of fluid called seroma, and weakened bones around the rib area being exposed to the radiation.

■ Endocrine Therapy

Endocrine therapy can significantly improve the prognoses of hormone receptor-positive breast cancer patients. Endocrine therapy drugs can be categorized as selective estrogen receptor modulators (SERM—for example, tamoxifen), aromatase inhibitors (such as letrozole and exemestane), or selective estrogen receptor degrader (SERD, such as fulvestrant). These drugs are designed to disrupt the growth of specific cancer cells; however, some patients do not respond to these treatments.

Drug Resistance. Drug resistance can be of two types, namely primary and secondary, in which the primary cells and tumors express hormone receptors, but they are not sensitive to endocrine therapy, whereas the secondary population responds to endocrine therapy initially and acquires resistance gradually with continued endocrine therapy. The mechanisms of drug resistance in endocrine therapy are complicated. It is not caused by a single factor, but a combination of multiple factors, which is also the reason for the poor therapeutic effect of drugs developed for a single factor in clinical practice. Currently, the mechanisms of endocrine therapy resistance in breast cancer have been found to include estrogen receptor gene abnormalities. More specifically, the incidence of ESR1 mutation in primary breast cancer is less than 1 percent, while it is more than 20 percent in aromatase inhibitor-resistant breast cancer patients.

New therapies, however, are now being examined to evaluate endocrine therapy resistance in hormone receptor-positive breast cancer patients. Endocrine therapy is the prominent strategy for the treatment of hormone-positive breast cancers. The emergence of resistance to endocrine therapy is a major health concern among hormone-positive breast cancer patients. Resistance to endocrine therapy demands the design of newer therapeutic strategies. The understanding of underlying molecular mechanisms of endocrine resistance, components of the tumor microenvironment (TME), and interaction of resistant breast cancer cells with the cellular/acellular components of the environment inside the tumor are essential to formulate new therapeutic strategies for the treatment of endocrine therapy-resistant breast cancers.

■ T-Cell Therapy

T-cell therapy, also known as *adoptive cell therapy*, is a branch of cancer immunotherapy that utilizes the immune cells to attack cancer cells. One of the first methods of immunotherapy created was cytokine therapy, which uses cytokines to activate certain immune cells to antitumor immunity. In addition, as you have seen, natural killer (NK) cells are an essential component of innate immunity and are critical in destroying tumor cells without prior stimulation with antigens. (See Chapter 8, "Strengthening Your Immune System," page 217 for more information.)

Chimeric antigen receptor (CAR) T-cell therapy represents a major advancement in personalized cancer treatment. In this form of therapy, a person's own T-cells are genetically engineered to express a synthetic receptor that binds a tumor antigen. CAR T-cells are then infused back into the patient's body to attack and destroy chemotherapy-resistant cancer. Moreover, accumulating evidence shows that the immune system itself plays a crucial role in the outcomes of some breast cancer subgroups, especially more aggressive, proliferative ones such as triple-negative and HER2-positive breast cancer. Tumor-infiltrating lymphocytes reflect the attempt of the host to eradicate malignancies, and during the last decades people with triple negative breast cancer (TNBC) and individuals with a high level of tumor-infiltrating lymphocytes (TILs such as CD4+, CD8+, and FOXP3+) have shown better short-term and long-term outcomes.

Consequently, some of these immunotherapies as well as the individual's own immunology have shown promising results on invasive or metastatic breast cancers, while others have shown an enhanced effect when used in conjunction with chemotherapy. Many of these immunotherapies are experimental and are in the process of clinical trials and show positive outcomes for the treatment of breast cancer.

■ Theragnostics

Theragnostics, also called *theranostics*, is a technique that uses radiopharmaceuticals (radioactive drugs) to detect and destroy cancer and other diseases. It has been used since the 1940s but is again gaining significant traction. Theragnostic is based on the binding of radionuclides to molecular targets. Therapeutic agents then attach to those specific markers found in or around diseased cells. They then emit signals that are picked up by PET scan, which reveal the location of the disease and deliver focused radiation that kills the cancer cells at the molecular level. Thus, this allows a personalized approach to patients with effective treatment and comparably small side effects.

CONCLUSION

As you have read in this chapter, there are different types of breast cancer. The type of breast cancer is based on which cells in the breast become cancerous. Knowing how your breast looks and feels and being aware of signs and symptoms can help you in detecting the cancer early and at a time when it is easiest to treat. Although ultrasound and mammography remain the most commonly used conventional methods of diagnosing breast cancer, other diagnostic tests, such as thermography, DCE-MRI, MRE, PET, PET-CT, SLNB, and BSGI are now being considered and used. The therapy your healthcare provider chooses depends on the type of breast cancer, and if it has metastasized.

Cancer treatments can have various side effects depending on the type of treatment given, the drugs or therapies used, and the woman's overall health. The next chapter discusses the therapies and prevention methods concerning possible side effects of cancer treatments.

2

Treating Cancer Therapy Side Effects

The truth is, fighting breast cancer might be the most difficult thing you ever have to do. It's a 24-hour-a-day ordeal that can drain both your brain and your body. Cancer can hit you on multiple fronts—the disease itself, the aggressive treatments used to fight it, and the side effects of those treatments. Dealing with all of this can take a real toll on you—both physically and mentally. There are many possible side effects of cancer therapies. The most common include swollen breasts, nausea, fatigue, and skin irritation. However, based on the chemotherapy drugs used, there can also be a number of other side effects—some serious, some mild. Treatment centers will normally provide you with medications to deal with these issues. However, don't be embarrassed to talk to your physician about what to expect prior to receiving the treatment or to ask for help during the process.

There are also a number of nutrients that can be of benefit in dealing with some of these side effects. Unfortunately, some of these can lead to more serious health issues. The three most common of these conditions are bone loss (*osteoporosis*), pains caused by nerve damage (*peripheral neuropathy*), and a weakened immune system.

Let's begin by first looking at some of these nutrients and what you can do to lessen or alleviate some of these stressors.

BREAST CANCER NUTRIENTS DURING CHEMOTHERAPY AND RADIATION

Some nutrients interfere with chemotherapy or radiation, or they may improve the course of your treatment. This section examines nutrients that have been shown to be helpful given in the right amounts during chemotherapy and/

or radiation. Not all healthcare providers agree on which nutrients can be used, so always check first with your doctor before beginning any nutritional therapy.

■ OMEGA-3 FATTY ACIDS (EPA and DHA)

There are a number of different omega-3 fatty acids. The two most important are *eicosapentaenoic acid* (EPA) and *docosahexaenoic acid* (DHA). They are essential in maintaining proper membrane function and they assist in circulation and oxygen uptake, reduce inflammation, and have many other functions in the body. (See page 50.) EPA and DHA have been reported to reduce breast cancer incidence. Animal and human studies have demonstrated that omega-3 fatty acids induce chemosensitization, which means that it effectively stops the growth of breast cancer cells. It works through several pathways from producing inflammation-resolving metabolites to protecting normal cells against toxic chemicals and so much more.

These effects have led to omega-3 fatty acids being tested as potential additions to traditional chemotherapy. In a small study, twenty-five metastatic breast cancer patients (pre- and postmenopausal; PR/ER positive and negative) treated with anthracycline-based chemotherapy have underlined safety and potential benefits of DHA supplementation. Data from this study reported increased disease-free survival. Furthermore, a slightly lower toxicity of chemotherapy regarding anemia, thrombopenia, and gastrointestinal toxicity has also been seen. Other studies have supported these results.

In addition, EPA and DHA are safe and effective in reducing the common chemotherapy-related side effects, such as bone density loss, peripheral neuropathy, and weight gain. There are also no negative effects on the heart. Loss of bone density and increased fracture rate are a side effect of cytotoxic chemotherapy in premenopausal women or of *aromatase inhibitors* (AI) in postmenopausal women. A small pilot trial suggested that four grams per day EPA plus DHA stopped bone reabsorption in postmenopausal women receiving aromatase inhibitors, a form of hormone therapy drugs that prevent and treat estrogen-related breast cancer in postmenopausal women. Moreover, a study demonstrated that omega-3 fatty acid supplementation in obese postmenopausal breast cancer patients treated with AI significantly reduced AI-associated joint pain. Cognitive and neurological side effects are also commonly seen in women undergoing chemotherapy.

Cancer patients experience impairments in attention, processing speed, executive function and working memory, depending on agents used, intensity and duration of treatment, and other predisposing disease processes. In fact, in a small-randomized trial, women with breast cancer who received pacli-taxel therapy EPA and DHA reduced the incidence of neuropathy from 60 percent to 30 percent. Interestingly, a diet high in sugar caused a reduction in the decreased neuroprotective effects of omega-3 fatty acids. Therefore, EPA and/or DHA may soon be recommended as adjuvants for chemotherapy and radiotherapy in individuals undergoing treatment for breast cancer.

■ GREEN TEA

Green tea is recognized for its wide range of medicinal benefits, which can be attributed to the many organic compounds it contains. The most signifi-cant of green tea's components is believed to be *epigallocatechin 3-gallate*, or EGCG. Epigallocatechin 3-gallate (EGCG), the main representative of *catechin* (a type of antioxidant found in plants, fruits, and vegetables), shows strong chemopreventive and chemotherapeutic effects against breast cancer. Exper-imental trials suggest the positive effects of EGCG with conventional cancer therapies, as well as improvement of possible related side effects due to its anti-inflammatory and antioxidant activities. Cell and animal studies reveal that EGCG hinders multiple signaling pathways. Additionally, EGCG can inhibit angiogenesis and tumor invasiveness, as well as change the immune system function. Studies have discovered that the combination of green tea catechins with tamoxifen or paclitaxel enhances treatment of both ER$^+$ and ER$^-$ breast cancer, improving the safety profile.

Two Japanese observational studies showed that consumption of a min-imum of five cups of green tea in breast cancer (BC) patients is associated with decreased risk of reoccurrence, especially in people with early stage (I and II) disease. No improvement was seen in patients with stage III or IV disease. In addition, a Chinese study (the Shanghai Breast Cancer Survival Study) demonstrated that tea intake (about three cups a day) during the first 60 months after cancer diagnosis is associated with improved survival among women with triple-negative breast cancer. In addition, due to their ability to decrease reactive oxygen species, green tea polyphenols can lower the adverse effects induced by chemotherapeutic agents. Preclinical trials have shown the beneficial effect of EGCG in reducing heart damage resulting from treatment with the medication doxorubicin.

ANTIOXIDANTS, VITAMINS, AND MINERALS

The use of vitamin and mineral supplements in cancer patients is very pop-ular because of their potential anticancer properties. They may also reduce oxidative damage triggered by chemotherapy and/or radiation. Observational data from the Lung Adjuvant Cisplatin Evaluation (LACE) study showed that 72 percent of breast cancer patients were self-prescribing multivitamins. Multivitamin use, along with a diet rich in fruits and vegetables and physical activity, may be beneficial in improving the prognosis of breast cancer. The controversial discussion regarding supplementation with antioxidant agents during cancer treatment is due mainly to their potential interaction with conventional cancer treatments. Since radiotherapy and many chemotherapeutic drugs (such as anthracyclines) exert their anticancer effects through reactive oxygen species (ROS) production, antioxidant agents may therefore reduce their efficacy protecting both normal and tumor cells from oxidative damage. Based on increasing evidence from phase II and III trials, the widespread use of antioxidants during chemo and radiation treatments is not yet convincing.

▓ CALCIUM

Some nutrients like calcium may be beneficial since calcium is needed for healthy bones, but it may also be detrimental since you may develop *hypercalcemia* (high calcium levels) when you have breast cancer. In fact, hypercalcemia of malignancy is quite common and affects about 44 percent of all patients that have cancer. Work with your healthcare provider to have your blood calcium levels checked on a regular basis.

▓ VITAMIN C

Vitamin C, or ascorbic acid, is a water-soluble vitamin involved in several biological processes. Vitamin C can induce *apoptosis* (death) of cancer cells and enhance immune response as shown in cell studies. However, the effects of vitamin C supplementation on breast cancer mortality or reoccurrence are controversial and may be dependent on dose, source of vitamin C, route of administration (oral versus intravenous), and timing and duration of supplementation. The association between vitamin C and vitamin E supplementation during chemotherapy with tamoxifen, in postmenopausal women with BC, has been demonstrated to restore an optimal antioxidant state. Similar findings have been obtained in studies on intravenous vitamin C administration. Your healthcare provider will run a blood study to check you for *glucose-6-phosphate dehydrogenase deficiency* (G6PD) before you receive IV vitamin C. Deficiency of G6PD may be due to mutations that change the protein structure and therefore reduce its activity, or the amount of enzyme produced. G6PD deficiency makes red cells highly vulnerable to oxidative damage and therefore susceptible to *hemolysis*, which damages the red blood cells.

VITAMIN D

In cancer, vitamin D has been demonstrated to regulate the expression of genes involved in cancer development and progression, stimulating cell differentiation and apoptosis or inhibiting cell proliferation, angiogenesis, invasion, inflammation, and metastatic potential. Vitamin D deficiency is common among individuals with breast cancer, and it is considered a negative prognostic factor. (See page 87 and page 206 for further discussion.) In addition, vitamin D supplementation has been shown to lessen joint pain and fatigue associated with letrozole treatment (an aromatase inhibitor). In breast patients whose bone density can be affected by chemotherapy-induced menopause and aromatase inhibitors, it is recommended that vitamin D and calcium both be taken, since vitamin D supplementation alone has reported no benefits for bone density or fracture risk.

VITAMIN E

Vitamin E is a group of eight fat-soluble vitamins—comprising four *tocopherols* (vitamin E) and four *tocotrienols* (primary form of vitamin E)—with antioxidant and anti-inflammatory properties. Studies are controversial as to whether vitamin E is beneficial or harmful during chemotherapy.

SELENIUM

Selenium is an antioxidant mineral that is crucial for the activity of antioxidant enzymes (for example, glutathione peroxidase), and which participates in the metabolism of oxidants and drugs. Usually, patients with breast cancer have significantly lower selenium levels. Selenium supplementation may reduce the side effects of conventional cytotoxic therapies (such as kidney toxicity by cisplatin, mucositis by radiotherapy) without affecting their antitumor efficacy. Oral mucositis, a condition causing inflammation and irritation of the mouth's tissue, is one of the most common, debilitating complications of cancer treatments, particularly chemotherapy and radiation. It can lead to several problems, including pain, nutritional deficiencies due to an inability to eat, and increased risk of infection due to open sores in the mouth. This is important since it helps improve compliance, decrease patients dropping out of cancer therapies, and also allows the use of higher possible dosages. However, selenium is *toxic* if taken in excess. Thus, selenium levels should be drawn before taking high-dose selenium as a supplement.

LOSS OF ZINC AND OTHER HEAVY METALS

Some chemotherapeutic drugs may cause a chelation process to occur that can cause some elimination of zinc and other heavy metals in your body, leading to zinc depletion and contributing to loss of taste. Studies have demonstrated that zinc supplementation may be beneficial for individuals undergoing cancer chemotherapy in improving taste perception. Dry mouth, which is also a possible side effect of chemotherapy, may be improved with the supplementation of zinc. One study revealed that the addition of zinc leads to better nutritional intake and helped individuals having chemotherapy maintain their weight.

OSTEOPOROSIS (BONE LOSS)

Your body's bones are designed to be strong enough to keep your body's structure in place—to protect your organs and allow you to be mobile. Normal bones have enough strength and density to do just that. Over time, however, the density of the bones may weaken. This condition is called *osteoporosis*. Osteoporosis is a skeletal disorder characterized by low bone mass and the deterioration of bone tissue. When it happens, bones become fragile and are more likely to fracture or break. If untreated, this disease can progress painlessly until a fracture occurs. The most common places people with osteoporosis experience fractures are the spine, the hip, and the wrists. Today, one in three postmenopausal women is likely to develop an osteoporotic fracture in one of these three places.

There are many reasons this can happen. Facts can include heredity, poor diet, lack of exercise, aging, and drugs—a host of drugs, including some used to fight breast cancer. Certain hormone-based drugs and chemotherapies have been shown to increase the risk of developing mild bone loss (*osteopenia*) and major bone loss (*osteoporosis*). Ask your doctor about the risk level for developing signs of osteoporosis based on the therapy you may be on. Also remember to have your own bone density measured before starting on one of these treatments to keep track of your bone's condition.

As you will see, there are a number of things you can do to protect yourself from developing this disease.

SYMPTOMS OF OSTEOPOROSIS

Because osteoporosis progression does not come with pain, it is not easy to detect. Its symptoms may appear only after a fracture has occurred. The following are symptoms associated with osteoporosis:

☐ Back pain. This may be due to a broken or collapsed vertebra in the spine.

☐ Bone fractures. A fracture may occur due to a fall or a trip down a step.

☐ Loss of an inch or more of your height. This may be due to compression of the spinal vertebrae.

☐ Changes in your posture. Finding yourself stooping or leaning forward more as you walk.

RISK FACTORS FOR OSTEOPOROSIS

Osteoporosis does not have a single cause. The many risk factors for developing osteoporosis include:

- Abnormal cortisol levels
- Alcohol abuse
- Calcium deficiency
- Chemotherapy
- Decrease in level of estrogen
- Electrolyte imbalance with low levels of potassium
- Excessive alcohol intake
- Excessive intake of vitamin A
- Excessive protein intake
- Excessive zinc supplementation
- Fluoride in drinking water
- High fat diets
- Hyperparathyroidism—too much activity in the parathyroid glands
- Hyperthyroidism—thyroid gland produces too much thyroid hormone
- Lack of exercise
- Menopause
- No menstrual cycle for more than 6 months prior to menopause
- Oxidative stress (with a negative influence on bone structure)
- Smoking
- Soft drink consumption
- Vitamin D deficiency
- Too much acid in your body. Acid-base imbalance is important. A diet higher in fruits and vegetables produces a more alkaline environment, which reduces urinary calcium excretion. Furthermore, whether a food is acidic or alkaline before it is eaten does not necessarily determine how it contributes to acid-base balance after it is eaten. Moreover, foods that are higher in sulfur amino acids, phosphorus, or chloride (for example: meat, grains, nuts, and dairy products) contribute to the acidic load. Likewise, foods that are potassium and magnesium salts of organic acids like fruits and vegetables contribute to the alkali load.

- Caffeine increases calcium loss. If an individual drinks three cups of coffee daily, they lose 45 mg of calcium. Coffee also contains twenty-nine different acids, which also draw calcium out of bones. In fact, more than 1,000 over-the-counter medications contain caffeine, including weight loss products, cold preparation, pain relievers, and allergy products.

- Genetic predisposition. It is also estimated that 50 percent to 80 percent of the individual variability in bone mass is determined by genetics, such as fair complexion and thin bone structure.

- Poor diet. The DASH (Dietary Approaches to Stop Hypertension) trial revealed that people who ate a diet higher in fruits and vegetables had lower bone turnover markers.

- Surgeries. Some surgeries increase the risk of bone loss including total thyroidectomy (complete removal of the thyroid gland) and removal of part or all of the intestines, including intestinal bypass surgery for weight control.

- Medications can also increase the risk of bone loss. The following are some of these medications:

  - Aromatase inhibitors
  - Corticosteroids
  - Cyclosporine
  - Dilantin and other anticonvulsants
  - Excessive thyroid medication
  - Gonadotropin-releasing hormone agonists
  - Heparin
  - Isoniazid
  - Lasix
  - Lithium
  - Long-term use of some antibiotics
  - Medroxyprogesterone
  - Methotrexate
  - PPIs (antacids)
  - SSRIs (antidepressants)
  - Tetracycline

MEDICAL CONDITIONS COMMONLY ASSOCIATED WITH OSTEOPOROSIS

The risk of osteoporosis is higher in women who have certain medical conditions, such as:

- Anorexia nervosa
- Celiac
- COPD
- Crohn's disease
- Cushing's disease
- Diabetes mellitus
- Fat malabsorption
- Gallbladder disease

- Chronic low back pain
- Numerous stress fractures
- Hypercalciuria
- Hypochlorhydria
- Kidney disease
- Lactose intolerance
- Multiple myeloma
- Nulliparous
- Primary biliary cirrhosis
- Rheumatoid arthritis
- Scoliosis

CONVENTIONAL THERAPIES FOR OSTEOPOROSIS

The following are conventional therapies for osteoporosis:

- Bisphosphonates are by far the most common conventional therapy for bone loss. The following are possible side effects of this class of drugs:

- Acute phase reaction (transient flu-like symptoms)
- Atrial fibrillation (irregular heartbeat)
- GI symptoms
- Hypocalcemia (low calcium level)
- Increase in hip fracture after five years of use
- Musculoskeletal pain
- Ocular (eye) side effects
- Osteonecrosis (deterioration) of the jawbone

- Parathyroid hormone (PTH) is FDA-approved to build bone. It is a prescription and is to be used for severe osteoporosis in postmenopausal women. It is not to be used for mild osteoporosis. In addition, it is not to be used for more than 24 months in the patient's lifetime. It is taken as a subcutaneous daily injection. Possible side effects include the following:

- Active Paget's disease (causes bones to grow larger and become weaker)
- Back spasms
- Depression
- Heartburn
- Increased risk of developing osteosarcoma (cancer of the bone).
- Itching, swelling, redness at site of injection
- Leg cramps
- Skeletal malignant conditions
- Unexplained elevations of alkaline phosphatase (blood study)

- Calcium (See pages 31–34 for more information on the use of calcium.)

PERSONALIZED THERAPIES FOR OSTEOPOROSIS

The following are personalized therapies for osteoporosis:

LIFESTYLE CHANGES

- Avoid acidic foods. (See *Acid-Creating Foods* inset below.)

- Decrease the amount of sugar in your diet. Sugar decreases the rate the body absorbs and increases the elimination of calcium and magnesium, which can lead to bone loss.

Acid-Creating Foods

The average American diet includes many foods that, once eaten, create acid in your body. If you eat mostly acidic foods and not enough alkaline foods, your body must find alkalizing materials elsewhere to neutralize its pH levels. It often must resort to using the calcium and protein in your bones. As a result, your bones can become weakened, possibly irrevocably, and your body systems can age at an accelerated pace, resulting in a slew of related problems. The following foods create particularly high acidity levels in your body:

- Chocolate
- Dairy products, such as butter, cheese, ice cream, milk, and yogurt
- Drinks, such as beer, black tea, coffee, and soft drinks
- Fish, such as haddock
- Fruit, such as blueberries, cranberries, and dried fruit
- Grains, such as barley, oats, rice, wheat, and white bread
- Honey
- Meat products, such as beef, chicken, ham, turkey, and veal
- Nuts, such as peanuts and walnuts
- Processed soybeans
- Sugar
- Vegetables, such as corn
- White vinegar

- Exercise (walking three to four times a week for 30 to 50 minutes).
- Reduce alcohol intake.
- Decrease stress. You can do all the things suggested in this section, but if you stay stressed, you may still break down bone!

NUTRIENTS

To maintain your bone health, your body needs calcium, magnesium, boron, zinc, copper, silicon, phosphorus, manganese, vitamins B_6, B_{12}, D, and K, folate, and strontium. Additionally, your body must have an optimal amount of bioflavonoids and amino acids to maintain and build bone.

▥ BORON

Boron, along with vitamin D, increases the mineral content in bone and also increases cartilage formation.

Food Sources

- Almonds
- Apples
- Broccoli
- Cauliflower
- Dates
- Grapes
- Green leafy vegetables, such as kale
- Hazelnuts
- Honey
- Legumes
- Peaches
- Peanuts
- Pears
- Prunes
- Raisins
- Tomatoes

▥ CALCIUM

Calcium is the most abundant mineral in the body. More than 99 percent of the body's calcium is in its bones and teeth. Calcium has many functions in the body, including the important role it plays in supporting bone and tooth structure. Calcium reduces bone loss and decreases bone turnover. Numerous studies have shown that calcium supplementation can help decrease bone loss by 30 to 50 percent. The recommended dose is 500 mg twice a day.

Important Facts About Calcium

- Calcium carbonate is not the best form of calcium to use. Calcium citrate or hydroxyapatite are now the preferred forms.
- Calcium intake helps lower cholesterol.

- Calcium is also needed for the absorption of vitamin B_{12}.

- Calcium should be taken throughout the day for maximum absorption because your body can only absorb 500 mg at a time. It is best taken with meals and at bedtime.

- Consuming chewable antacid tablets is not a good way to intake calcium, due to poor absorption.

- Hydrochloric acid, citric acid, glycine, and lysine all help increase calcium absorption.

- Magnesium aids calcium absorption by converting vitamin D into its active form.

- Milk is not the best source of calcium since pasteurization destroys up to 32 percent of the available calcium.

- Use only pharmaceutical-grade calcium supplements. Lower grade products may be contaminated with lead, mercury, arsenic, aluminum, or cadmium. (For suggestions on companies that use pharmaceutical-grade supplements, see the *Resources* section on page 285.)

- Vitamin C increases calcium absorption by 100 percent.

- You can take too much calcium.

Factors That Decrease Calcium Absorption

- Aging process
- Caffeine
- Celiac disease
- Chronic alcoholism
- Cigarette smoking (nicotine)
- Glucocorticoid excess
- Hyperthyroidism
- Hypoparathyroidism
- Malabsorptive bariatric surgery
- Menopause
- Oxalate
- Phytate or phytic acid (found in seeds, grains, and beans)
- Sugar
- Vitamin D deficiency
- Obesity

Factors That Increase Calcium Absorption

- B-cell lymphoma and other active cancers
- Carbohydrates
- Crohn's disease

- Estrogen
- Fat
- Food
- Growth
- Lactation
- Lactose
- Lysine
- Prebiotics
- Pregnancy
- Primary hyperparathyroidism
- Probiotics
- Protein
- Sarcoidosis
- Tuberculosis (TB)
- Vitamin D

Excessive calcium consumption or elevated calcium levels due to a disease process may have negative effects, such as:

- Blocks the uptake of manganese in the body
- Causes kidney stones
- Clogs arteries (predisposes to heart disease)
- Decreases iron absorption
- Decreases thyroid function
- Interferes with the absorption of magnesium
- Interferes with the absorption of zinc
- Interferes with the making of vitamin K

Additionally, calcium supplementation can interact with medications. It increases the toxicity of digoxin (a heart medication) and decreases the absorption of the antibiotics—for example, ciprofloxacin and fluoroquinolone. Calcium can also inhibit the absorption of tetracycline, another antibiotic.

Food Sources

- Almonds
- Barley
- Beet greens
- Black beans
- Bluefish
- Brazil nuts
- Brick cheese
- Broccoli
- Chicken
- Chinese cabbage
- Dandelion greens
- Dates
- Eggs
- English walnuts
- Garbanzo beans
- Ground beef
- Halibut
- Hazelnuts
- Kale
- Kelp
- Mackerel
- Mustard greens
- Olives, ripe
- Parsley
- Pecans
- Pinto beans
- Prunes, dried
- Rice, brown
- Salmon
- Sesame seeds

- Shrimp
- Soybeans
- Sunflower seeds
- Tofu
- Turnip greens
- Watercress
- White beans
- Yogurt

When you're looking to increase your calcium, there are a few things you should avoid. The items on the following list all decrease calcium absorption.

Foods That Decrease Calcium Absorption

- Cocoa, chocolate
- Diet high in breads
- Excessive zinc supplementation
- High fat diet
- High fiber cereals, fiber supplements (wait two hours after eating before taking calcium)
- Rhubarb
- Soft drinks
- Spinach
- Swiss chard
- White flour
- Whole wheat

■ COPPER

Copper should be supplemented if zinc is supplemented. Copper and zinc must sit in appropriate ratios in the body. Usually, 10 to 15 milligrams (mgs) of zinc to one milligram of copper are needed. Copper plays an important role in bone metabolism and turnover.

Food Sources

- Almonds
- Barley
- Beef liver
- Brazil nuts
- Buckwheat
- Butter
- Carrots
- Clams
- Coconut
- Cod liver oil
- Garlic
- Hazelnuts
- Lamb chops
- Olive oil
- Oysters
- Peanuts
- Pecans
- Pork loin
- Rye grain
- Shrimp
- Split peas, dry
- Sunflower oil
- Walnuts

■ MAGNESIUM

Magnesium has 300 functions in the body. It is very much needed for bone health. The following are roles magnesium plays in bone health. The recommended dose is 400 to 600 mg a day.

- Activates bone-building osteoblasts (cells that form bone tissue)

- Activates vitamin D

- Aids in parathyroid function (decreases bone breakdown)

- Helps calcitonin function (increases the absorption of calcium)

- Increases mineralization density

- Increases the absorption of calcium

Causes of Magnesium Deficiency

- Alcoholism

- Antibiotics (gentamicin, carbenicillin, or amphotericin B)

- Asthma medications (beta-agonists or epinephrine)

- Caffeine intake

- Cyclosporine, which prevents organ transplant rejection

- Diarrhea

- Digoxin use (heart medication)

- Diuretics (water pills)

- Drugs used for chemotherapy (cisplatinum, vinblastine, or bleomycin)

- Excessive fiber intake

- Excessive sugar intake

- Extreme athletic competition

- Foods high in oxalic acid (almonds, cocoa, spinach, tea)

- Laxatives

- Phosphates in soft drinks

- Steroids

- Stress

- Surgery

- Trans fatty acids

- Trauma

Food Sources

- Almonds
- Apricots, dried
- Avocados
- Brazil nuts
- Buckwheat
- Cashews
- Cheddar cheese
- Coconut
- Collard leaves
- Corn
- Dandelion greens

- Dark green vegetables
- Dates
- Figs, dried
- Kelp
- Parsley
- Peanuts
- Prunes, dried
- Pumpkin seeds
- Rice, brown
- Rye

- Sesame seeds
- Shrimp
- Soybeans
- Spinach, raw
- Sunflower seeds
- Swiss chard
- Tofu
- Wheat bran
- Wheat germ
- Wheat grain
- Yeast, brewer's

■ MANGANESE

Manganese is needed for the repair of soft bone and connective tissue and is used for bone growth and maintenance. Excessive calcium supplementation can decrease the absorption of manganese. The recommended dose is two milligrams (mg) a day. Manganese is commonly contained in your multivitamin.

Food Sources

- Avocados
- Bay leaves
- Brazil nuts
- Buckwheat
- Cloves
- Ginger
- Hazelnuts
- Oatmeal
- Pecans
- Seaweed
- Tea
- Thyme
- Whole wheat

■ PHOSPHORUS

Phosphorus regulates bone formation, inhibits bone re-absorption, and affects the regulation of calcium. Most Americans eat enough phosphorus-containing foods that low phosphorus levels are rarely seen.

Food Sources

- Almonds
- Beef liver
- Brazil nuts
- Brewer's yeast
- Brown rice
- Cashews
- Cheddar cheese
- Chicken
- Dried pinto beans
- Dried soybeans
- Eggs
- English walnuts
- Garlic
- Hulked sesame seeds
- Kelp
- Millet
- Peanuts
- Pearled barley
- Pecans
- Pumpkin seeds
- Rye grain
- Scallops
- Squash seeds
- Sunflower seeds
- Wheat
- Wheat bran
- Wheat germ

■ SILICON

Silicon is a trace mineral that has been shown to increase bone mineral density. It is found in many forms, but the only form that is useful to humans is *orthosilicic acid*. Foods that are high in fiber usually contain silicon. The recommended dose is one to five milligrams (mg) a day. High dosages can cause kidney stone production.

Food Sources

- Apples
- Celery
- Cherries
- Endive

- Legumes
- Oats
- Onions
- Oranges

- Rice bran
- Root vegetables
- Unrefined grains

STRONTIUM

Strontium, in the form of strontium ranelate, is a wonderful trace mineral that promotes bone formation and decreases bone resorption. Studies found a reduction in vertebral fractures of 37 percent and 40 percent, and a reduction in non-vertebral fractures of 14 percent and 16 percent.

VITAMIN B_6, B_{12}, AND FOLATE

Levels of vitamins B_6, B_{12}, and folate are commonly low in individuals with osteoporosis. Low levels of these nutrients are associated with elevated homocysteine levels. High homocysteine levels interfere with collagen cross-linking, which leads to a defective bone matrix. This may be since high amounts of homocysteine are associated with vitamin B_{12} deficiency and poor methylation, which is a major risk factor for breast cancer. Therefore, people with elevated homocysteine levels have an increased risk of developing osteoporosis. B vitamins commonly become low when you are stressed. They are water soluble and must be taken twice a day. Discuss with your healthcare provider the possibility of having a homocysteine test done and if you should be taking methylated B vitamins or not.

VITAMIN D

Vitamin D is a prohormone—that is, it is a precursor to the hormone *calcitriol*, which has many functions in the body.

- Calcitriol (a hormonally active form of vitamin D) has been shown to be a powerful regulator of mineral metabolism. It increases the concentration of calcium and phosphate in the plasma. Calcitriol also has a direct effect on bone resorption since it acts as a calcium-regulating hormone.

- A study concluded that vitamin D supplementation decreased the risk of vertebral fractures by 37 percent and non-vertebral fractures by 23 percent.

- In another trial, vitamin D supplementation reduced the relative risk of hip fracture by 26 percent and any non-vertebral fracture by 23 percent compared to taking calcium alone or a placebo.

- A study showed a link between deficient levels of vitamin D and premature aging of bone.

- Optimal vitamin D status: 55 to 80 nanograms per milliliter (ng/mL). Also get a calcium level. If calcium levels are elevated, find the cause of the high level. Vitamin D excess alone is rarely the case.

- 25-OH vitamin D is currently the main indicator of how much vitamin D is in the body. It reflects vitamin D produced inside the body and that obtained from foods and supplements. Levels may be normal in patients who are vitamin D toxic and have high calcium levels due to vitamin D hypersensitivity syndrome. Hypersensitivity syndrome is commonly seen in the following cases:

  - Cancer
  - Crohn's disease
  - Granulomatous diseases
  - Hyperparathyroidism
  - Sarcoidosis
  - Tuberculosis

Diseases Associated With Low Vitamin D Levels

Optimal supplementation should be with vitamin D_3, not vitamin D_2.

- Ankylosing spondylitis
- Back pain
- Breast cancer
- Migraine headaches
- Multiple sclerosis (MS)
- Osteoarthritis
- Parkinson's disease
- Polycystic Ovary Syndrome (PCOS)
- Rheumatoid arthritis

Vitamin D is available mainly through sunlight. You make it in your skin from exposure to the sun. Topical sunscreens block vitamin D production by 97 to 100 percent. Dairy products, fish and fish liver oils, liver, sweet potatoes, and dandelion greens also contain some vitamin D. Supplementation with vitamin D is best done with vitamin D_3. New studies have shown that you may need more vitamin D than healthcare providers previously thought. Therefore, it is very important to have your vitamin D levels measured regularly to determine the perfect dose for you.

▓ VITAMIN K

Vitamin K has six major purposes in the body and there are three forms of vitamin K that the body can take in from diet. Twenty-five percent of your vitamin K comes from what you eat. Seventy-five percent of vitamin K used by the body is produced in our intestinal tract by friendly bacteria.

- K_1 (*phylloquinone*): found in leafy green vegetables, such as broccoli, Brussels sprouts, spinach, and turnip greens.

- K_2 (*menaquinone*): found in fermented soybeans and other fermented foods.

- K_3 (*menadione*): a synthetically produced form of vitamin K.

- K_7 (*menaquinone*): found in fermented soybeans and other fermented foods.

Causes of Vitamin K Deficiency

- Consumption of medications that cause malabsorption of fat

- Hydrogenated fat intake

- Lack of adequate beneficial bacteria in the intestine

- Lack of dietary intake

- Use of broad-spectrum antibiotics

- Vitamin K is important for bone mineralization. Osteocalcin is a key-protein for bone health and metabolic diseases. It is dependent on vitamin K to be produced. Low levels of vitamin K impair activation of osteocalcin and decrease the activity of bone-forming cells. Therefore, a low intake of vitamin K has been associated with bone loss. The good news is that vitamin K supplementation has been effective in preventing and treating osteoporosis.

- A recent study has shown that daily vitamin K intake must be at least 100 micrograms to maintain optimal bone health.

- Low bone density has been found in people treated with warfarin (a blood thinner). There is an association between fracture risk and warfarin use. Studies have shown a benefit and the safety of patients taking warfarin and low-dose vitamin K (100 micrograms a day).

Dosages of Vitamin K to Take

For those who are healthy, take 10 to 45 mg a day. Compared to vitamin K_1, K_{2-7} (a special form of vitamin K_2) is better absorbed and stays in the body longer. The half-life is three days, compared to a few hours for other forms of vitamin K. Vitamin K_{2-7} has been shown to have health benefits in bone loss, heart disease, cancer, Alzheimer's disease, diabetes, and peripheral neuropathy from all causes including chemotherapy. It also decreases inflammation.

Food Sources

- Asparagus
- Beef
- Broccoli
- Cheese
- Egg yolks
- Green beans
- Green cabbage

- Ham
- Lettuce
- Liver (beef, pork, chicken)
- Oats
- Peaches
- Potatoes

- Raisins
- Spinach
- Tomatoes
- Turnip greens
- Watercress
- Whole wheat

If you are on an anticoagulant (blood thinner) such as Coumadin, consult your doctor as to how much vitamin K-rich foods or supplementation you may need. Studies have revealed that bone density is reduced in some patients who take Coumadin. Likewise, an increased risk of bone fracture has been associated with long-term use of Coumadin. As previously discussed, research has shown that taking Coumadin with a low dose of vitamin K (100 micrograms a day) can be beneficial and safe. Still, you should consult your healthcare practitioner before beginning vitamin K supplementation if you are taking Coumadin.

A recent study also revealed that the supplementation of vitamin K_2 improves the effectiveness of bisphosphonates, which are medications used to treat osteoporosis.

■ ZINC

Zinc is used in many enzymatic reactions in the body. In fact, 100 enzymes use zinc as a cofactor in order to carry out their functions properly. It is needed for the formation of bones and skin.

Symptoms of Zinc Deficiency

- ☐ Acne
- ☐ Anemia
- ☐ Anorexia
- ☐ Arthritis
- ☐ Behavioral disturbances
- ☐ Brittle nails
- ☐ Craving sugary foods

- ☐ Dandruff
- ☐ Decreased ability to taste
- ☐ Decreased desire for protein-rich foods
- ☐ Decreased sense of smell
- ☐ Decreased sexual function

- ☐ Delayed sexual maturation
- ☐ Diarrhea
- ☐ Eczema
- ☐ Fatigue
- ☐ Frontal headaches
- ☐ Growth retardation
- ☐ Hair loss
- ☐ Immune deficiencies

- ☐ Impaired nerve conduction
- ☐ Impaired wound healing
- ☐ Impotence
- ☐ Infertility
- ☐ Low sperm count
- ☐ Memory impairment
- ☐ Negative nitrogen balance
- ☐ Nerve damage
- ☐ Night blindness
- ☐ Poor appetite
- ☐ Psoriasis
- ☐ Reduced salivation
- ☐ Sleep disturbances
- ☐ Stretch marks
- ☐ White spots on nails

Factors That Can Predispose You to a Zinc Deficiency

- ☐ Aging (zinc absorption decreases with age)
- ☐ AIDS
- ☐ Alcoholism
- ☐ Anorexia nervosa
- ☐ Caffeinated beverages
- ☐ Calcium supplementation
- ☐ Celiac disease
- ☐ Certain medications, such as: Cortisone, some diuretics (water pills), Tetracycline
- ☐ Chronic renal (kidney) failure
- ☐ Cirrhosis
- ☐ Cystic fibrosis
- ☐ Excess copper
- ☐ Food rich in phytic acid, such as unleavened bread, raw beans, seeds, nuts, and grains
- ☐ Hemolytic anemia
- ☐ Infection
- ☐ Inflammatory bowel disease
- ☐ Iron supplementation
- ☐ Nephritic syndrome
- ☐ Pancreatic insufficiency
- ☐ Pancreatitis
- ☐ Rheumatoid arthritis
- ☐ Short bowel syndrome
- ☐ Smoking
- ☐ Surgery
- ☐ Teas containing tannin

Food Sources

- Almonds
- Beef
- Black pepper
- Brazil nuts
- Buckwheat
- Chicken
- Chili powder
- Cinnamon
- Egg yolk
- Ginger root
- Ground round steak
- Hazelnuts
- Lamb chops
- Lima beans
- Milk, dry; non-fat
- Mustard
- Oats
- Oysters, fresh
- Paprika
- Peanuts
- Pecans

- Rye
- Sardines
- Soy lecithin
- Split peas
- Thyme
- Walnuts
- Whole wheat

KEEPING TRACK OF YOUR HEALTH

- See a Personalized Medicine specialist to have your hormones replaced if they are low and you are a candidate for hormone replacement. Estrogen replacement therapy has been shown to help build bone structure and to help maintain bone. Progesterone also helps build bone. A new study suggested that progesterone is effective to prevent and treat bone loss. Furthermore, testosterone not only builds bone but also improves the strength of bone. Yet another study revealed that transcutaneous (on the skin) hormone therapy with micronized estradiol and progesterone is the treatment of choice in postmenopausal osteoporosis, as evidenced by bone mineral density and biochemical markers.

- GI health. If your gut is not healthy, it is hard to absorb the minerals and other nutrients you need to build bone. Likewise, imbalances of microbiome (the collection of microorganisms) that live in your gastrointestinal tract can decrease absorption of minerals. Have your healthcare provider order a gut health test to determine the health of your GI tract. If your gut is not healthy, your healthcare provider will implement the 5-R program for gut restoration.

SUMMARY

Fractures connected to this bone-weakening condition can be life-altering. Fortunately, as you have seen, there are many therapies that can be used to prevent and treat bone loss which is a common potential side effect of breast cancer treatment. Talk with your healthcare provider to ascertain whether you need treatment, and which option is best for you.

PERIPHERAL NEUROPATHY (CIPN) INDUCED BY CHEMOTHERAPY

Various forms of chemotherapy can damage nerves outside the brain and spinal cord. This damage can make it difficult for the nerves to send and receive messages from the central nervous system. It is estimated that between twenty to thirty million people in the United States are thought to have peripheral neuropathy. Chances of it happening increases as adults age—45 and older.

It is estimated that about 30 percent to 40 percent of cancer patients experience this form of neuropathy after taking chemotherapy.

SYMPTOMS OF CIPN

Peripheral neuropathy is a nerve issue associated with the following symptoms:

☐ Numbness ☐ Prickling ☐ Burning pain

☐ Tingling ☐ Weakness

The incidence of peripheral neuropathy increases dramatically with age. Chemotherapy-induced peripheral neuropathy (CIPN) is a common dose-limiting side effect experienced by people receiving treatment for cancer. There is a considerable range of severity between patients.

Symptoms of CIPN typically begin during the first two months of treatment. These symptoms progress while chemotherapy continues. They then stabilize soon after treatment is completed. While most CIPN occurs related to the dose of medication, other drug-specific features may be present such as acute neurotoxicity. This can result in symptoms occurring from a single dose or the worsening after the chemo has been discontinued.

CAUSES OF CIPN

The following are known causes of peripheral neuropathy. Prior to making the diagnosis of CIPN in patients with cancer, it is important to consider all causes of possible neuropathy. It is important to also point out that 50% of the causes of peripheral neuropathy are unknown.

- AIDS
- Alcoholism
- Antiretrovirals
- Autoimmune diseases
- Chemotherapy-induced
- Diabetes (See *Diabetes and Nerve Damage* inset on page 44.)
- Exposure to toxins

- Hypothyroidism due to a deficiency of nutrients: Vitamins B_1, B_3, B_6, folic acid, B_{12}, E
- Inherited
- Medications
- 5-Azacytidine
- 5-Fluorouracil
- Amiodarone
- Renal failure (kidney failure)
- Viral and bacterial infections

Diabetes and Nerve Damage

Peripheral neuropathy is believed to occur in 40 to 60 percent of people with diabetes that have had it for 25 years or more. Diabetes is the most common cause of peripheral neuropathy. There are many pathophysiological factors that are associated with diabetic neuropathy including an increase in oxidative stress (too many free radicals and not enough antioxidants to get rid of them) and an increase in homocysteine which increases the risk of developing breast cancer, to name a few. Importantly, people with diabetes mellitus (metabolic disease involving elevated blood glucose levels) may be at a greater risk of developing peripheral neuropathy from chemotherapy.

CONVENTIONAL THERAPIES FOR CIPN

Conventional treatments for chemotherapy-induced peripheral neuropathy can include medications and non-medications. Here are the pharmacological treatments. (See page 45 for personalized non-medication treatments.)

- Analgesics (pain control medications)
- Anticonvulsant medications
- Non-steroidal anti-inflammatory drugs (NSAIDs)
- Topical capsaicin cream (topical analgesic)
- Treat underlying cause
- Tricyclic antidepressants

PERSONALIZED THERAPIES FOR CIPN

Personalized therapies have been found to be very successful for the treatment of peripheral neuropathy, no matter the cause. They include the following:

TRADITIONAL THERAPIES

- Acupuncture
- Botanicals and herbal therapies
- Tai chi

NON-INVASIVE THERAPIES

- Bioelectromagnetics
- Biofeedback

- Compounded transdermal pain control gel
- Infrared therapy

LIFESTYLE CHANGES

- Diet
- Exercise

NUTRIENTS

- Acetyl-L-Carnitine
- Alpha-lipoic acid
- Cobalamin (Vitamin B_{12})
- Evening primrose oil (EPO)
- Folate (Vitamin B_9)
- L-Glutamine
- Niacin (Vitamin B_3)
- Omega-3 fatty acids (EPA/DHA)
- Pantothenic Acid (Vitamin B_5)
- Pyridoxine (Vitamin B_6)
- Thiamine (Vitamin B_1)
- Vitamin E
- Vitamin K_{2-7}

TRADITIONAL THERAPIES

ACUPUNCTURE

Acupuncture and electroacupuncture have been found to be beneficial for peripheral neuropathy due to any of the following: diabetic, HIV-associated, chemotherapy-induced, and mixed origin. In numerous studies (some controlled and some not), acupuncture was shown to improve nerve conduction velocity, decrease numbness and pain by 66 percent to 87 percent. Also, symptoms were more improved using acupuncture for chemotherapy-induced peripheral neuropathy than by administering conventional therapies.

BOTANICALS AND HERBAL THERAPIES

Botanical and herbal therapies have been shown to improve peripheral neuropathy from various causes. For example, curcumin was shown to reduce diabetic neuropathic pain.

- Geranium oil as Neuragen PN has been shown in clinical trials to help with peripheral neuropathy. It is a mixture of five essential oils and six homeopathic ingredients. A multicenter, double-blind crossover study and a double-blind, randomized, placebo-controlled trial found that 93 percent of patients had a significant reduction in neuropathic pain within 30 minutes of application, which lasted up to 8 hours. The dose is one to two drops to put onto the affected area up to four times a day. If the skin is very sensitive, or if the area affected is wide, dilute four to five drops in one tablespoon of grape seed oil before applying. Avoid contact with eyes and open sores—and if a rash occurs, discontinue use.

TAI CHI

Conduction velocity—a slower-speed exercise (often caused by nerve damage) in which an electronic signal moves through a nerve—can lead to symptoms such as weakness, numbness, tingling, and impaired motor control. Studies have shown that gentle tai chi exercises improved peripheral nerve conduction velocities.

NON-INVASIVE THERAPIES

BIOELECTROMAGNETIC

Bioelectromagnetic therapy is the use of magnets hooked up to an electronic control, creating a bioelectronics force to affect the body's own internal electrical system. A double-blind, placebo-controlled, multicenter, randomized study showed that patients with diabetic peripheral neuropathy, stage II or III, who constantly wore static magnetic (450G) shoe soles for four months had significant reductions in their symptoms.

BIOFEEDBACK

This is a mind-body method that can help people learn to control their involuntary bodily functions—from breathing to muscle tension to heart rate. Biofeedback has been shown to reduce the pain associated with diabetic neuropathy.

COMPOUNDED TRANSDERMAL PAIN CONTROL GELS

Your Personalized Medicine practitioner can write a prescription for a compounded pain control gel that is also an effective treatment. If your doctor is not familiar with compounding, have them contact your local compounding pharmacist for pain control gel prescription suggestions. This therapy has been shown to be very valuable in many individuals.

▦ INFRARED THERAPY

This is a light-based treatment that uses infrared light to penetrate the skin to help relieve peripheral neuropathy as well as pain, inflammation, and other health issues.

LIFESTYLE CHANGES

▦ DIET

There are several dietary therapies that have been shown to be effective. Gluten sensitivity may be associated with peripheral neuropathy. Try avoiding all gluten to see if it is helpful. In addition, food allergies that are not associated with gluten may be a cause of peripheral neuropathy. See your Personalized Medicine practitioner for functional allergy testing. Avoiding all foods you are allergic to may help with this disease process.

Moreover, a case history showed a patient developed peripheral neuropathy from *monosodium glutamate* (MSG). Stop all MSG exposure and see if this is beneficial. Furthermore, aspartame may also be a culprit. There are some suggestions in case reports that peripheral neuropathy may be due to aspartame use. Controlled trials need to be done. Consider discontinuing aspartame use.

Tight control of blood sugar has been shown to decrease the incidence of diabetic neuropathy by up to 64 percent. If your blood sugar is elevated, you may have peripheral neuropathy secondary to elevated blood sugar, which can be compounded by your cancer treatment. As you will see, tightly controlling your blood sugar helps prevent breast cancer as well as aids in the prevention of a reoccurrence.

▦ EXERCISE

Research has shown that strengthening exercises, when done regularly, help to improve muscle strength in patients with peripheral neuropathy.

NUTRIENTS

Since nutritional depletion is a cause of this disease, consider replenishing the following nutrients that have been shown in the medical literature to be beneficial to treat peripheral neuropathy.

■ ACETYL-L-CARNITINE

This nutrient has been shown to help with symptoms of drug-induced peripheral neuropathy, particularly related to chemotherapy. A double-blind study of over 400 patients with peripheral neuropathy due to any cause were treated with acetyl-L-carnitine. Improvement was seen in some of the patients when acetyl-L-carnitine was used intramuscularly or by mouth.

In another study—which was a one-year randomized, double-blind, placebo-controlled study—it showed that acetyl-L-carnitine helped with the pain, nerve regeneration, and vibratory perception in individuals with neuropathy related to diabetes. In yet another trial, acetyl-L-carnitine was found to be beneficial for peripheral neuropathy in people with both type I and type II diabetes. It was more beneficial for type II form. The dose was 500 mg orally twice a day to 1,000 mg three times a day. Pain control was found to be better in higher doses. This dose is for individuals with normal kidney function.

■ ALPHA-LIPOIC ACID

Several randomized, double-blind, placebo-controlled trials have shown alpha-lipoic acid to help with peripheral and autonomic diabetic neuropathy. It has also been shown to be beneficial in patients with peripheral neuropathy secondary to chemotherapy and neuropathy that is toxin-induced. The dose is 600 to 1,800 mg a day. This dosage should only be used with your healthcare provider's instruction, since doses at 600 mg and above daily can cause your thyroid not to function optimally. It can negatively affect the conversion of T3 to the less active T4.

Consequently, your doctor will need to order your thyroid studies periodically. If you are diabetic, you may need to decrease the dose of your medication since lipoic acid helps to improve your blood sugar at doses of 300 mg and above. Make sure you check your blood sugar frequently. Contact your healthcare provider for a change in the dose of your medication if you notice your blood sugar is becoming too low.

■ COBALAMIN (VITAMIN B$_{12}$)

One of the symptoms of B$_{12}$ deficiency is peripheral neuropathy. A delay in treatment may cause irreversible neurological damage. Blood B$_{12}$ levels may be low normal and still the B$_{12}$ deficient peripheral neuropathy will respond to treatment. B$_{12}$ deficiency can occur without anemia or macrocytosis (enlarged red blood cells). You have macrocytosis if your MCV (measurement of size and volume of red blood cells) value on your blood count test is more than 100 femtoliters (fL). If you have an elevated serum (blood) methylmalonic acid (produced when amino acids break down) level and/or a high homocysteine level, it suggests a possible B_{12} deficiency.

Diabetic patients with neuropathy—in a small, double-blinded, placebo-controlled study—were treated with methyl cobalamin 500 micrograms three times a day. They showed improvement. Your doctor will suggest that you supplement with both B_{12} and folate if you have peripheral neuropathy.

■ EVENING PRIMROSE OIL (EPO)

This is a good source of omega-6 fatty acids, mostly as GLA (gamma-linolenic acid) and linoleic acid, which are both part of myelin and neuronal cell membranes. In fact, EPO may help prevent diabetic neuropathy. Studies have shown that supplementing with GLA increases the production of PGE1 (smooth muscle relaxant) by bypassing the blocked enzyme delta-6-desaturase that is commonly seen in people with hyperglycemia.

A randomized controlled trial showed that GLA aids in diabetic neuropathy. The dose is 360 mg daily of GLA as EPO. EPO may increase the effectiveness of some chemotherapeutic agents, as well as ceftazidime and cyclosporine. It may interact with phenothiazines (a class of drugs used to treat some mental and physical conditions) and increase the risk of seizures. Do not use EPO if you are taking a blood thinner. Non-steroidal anti-inflammatory drugs may counteract the effectiveness of EPO. Contact your doctor or pharmacist concerning other possible drug interactions.

■ FOLATE (VITAMIN B_9)

Peripheral neuropathy may be a manifestation of folate deficiency. It can occur without anemia or when red blood cells are larger than normal (*macrocytosis*). Consider supplementing with folate and B_{12} if you have peripheral neuropathy.

■ L-GLUTAMINE

L-glutamine has been shown to decrease the severity of the peripheral neuropathy caused by chemotherapy, as well as help prevent chemotherapy-induced neuropathy.

■ NIACIN (VITAMIN B_3)

In a case study, an alcoholic patient with peripheral neuropathy improved after taking vitamin B_3. This person had not previously responded to the thiamine. When you take B vitamins, take a B complex twice a day so that you receive the benefit from all of the B vitamins.

■ OMEGA-3 FATTY ACIDS (EPA/DHA)

These fatty acids are commonly known as fish oil. In a study of participants with diabetic neuropathy taking 1,800 mg of EPA a day for 48 weeks, they showed improvement in peripheral neuropathy symptoms. Do not take doses above 300 mg a day of EPA/DHA if you are taking a blood thinner.

■ PANTOTHENIC ACID (VITAMIN B$_5$)

In a case study, an individual that abused alcohol had peripheral neuropathy that responded to pantothenic acid and had not previously responded to thiamine alone.

■ PYRIDOXINE (VITAMIN B$_6$)

A deficiency has been shown to cause peripheral neuropathy in patients receiving some medication, such as isoniazid, amitriptyline, and hydralazine. B$_6$ deficiency is found in 50 percent of people that abuse alcohol.

■ THIAMINE (VITAMIN B$_1$)

Individuals at risk of developing a thiamine deficiency may develop peripheral neuropathy. Have your healthcare provider measure your thiamine level and replace it, if needed. Magnesium is needed for thiamine to work, so symptoms of thiamine deficiency may not respond to thiamine unless magnesium is included. *Benfotiamine* is the lipid-soluble derivative of B$_1$. It has been found in some trials to be better absorbed than the water-soluble forms. Studies have shown benfotiamine to improve neuropathy and increase nerve conduction velocity. The dose of benfotiamine is 150 to 300 mg twice a day for peripheral neuropathy.

■ VITAMIN E

Severe deficiency of vitamin E can cause peripheral neuropathy and other neurological symptoms. Peripheral neuropathy caused by chemotherapeutic agents may also improve with vitamin E. The dose is large, 800 to 1,600 IU a day. Vitamin E is a blood thinner and should not be used in high doses if you are taking a prescription blood thinner.

■ VITAMIN K2-7

In a trial, vitamin K$_{2-7}$ was shown to be beneficial for individuals with peripheral neuropathy due to B$_{12}$ deficiency and/or diabetes. The dose of K$_{2-7}$ is 100 micrograms a day. If you are taking a prescription blood thinner, contact your doctor before taking this nutrient.

SUMMARY

There are many different causes of peripheral neuropathy, some of which can be treated in different ways. Unlike most other types of pain, neuropathic pain does not usually get better with common painkillers, such as paracetamol and ibuprofen. As you have seen in this chapter, there are many conventional medicine treatments along with many personalized therapies that are effective to treat peripheral neuropathy.

WEAKENED IMMUNE SYSTEM

Breast cancer is one of the most common cancers in women, with the capability to spread to secondary organs. The ability to metastasize is the main cause of cancer-related deaths. Understanding how breast tumors progress is essential for developing better treatment strategies against breast cancer.

Until recently, it has been considered that breast cancer elicits a small immune response. However, science reveals that breast tumor progression is either prevented by the action of antitumor immunity or made worse by proinflammatory cytokines (proteins that control growth and activity) released mainly by the immune cells. Some types of cancer, such as melanoma, bladder, and renal cell carcinoma, have demonstrated a durable response to immunotherapeutic intervention. However, it is not the case with breast cancer. The causes of breast cancer's immune silence derive from methods that diminish immune recognition and others that promote strong suppression of your immune system. It is the mechanisms of immune evasion in breast cancers that are poorly defined.

Cancer immunosurveillance is an important process by which the immune system can monitor, recognize, and eliminate new tumor cells. There are three essential phases to this process which are elimination, equilibrium, and escape. Initially, both the innate and adaptive immune responses are able to control tumor growth. (See Chapter 8, "Strengthening Your Immune System," for a comprehensive discussion of how your immune system works.)

In the elimination phase, innate and adaptive immunity work together to detect and destroy transformed cells or cancer cells before they are observed clinically. Upon maturation, tumor cells and the immune system enter an equilibrium that keeps the tumor growth under control. During this phase of equilibrium, if another cycle of immune responses is unable to eliminate the new cancer cells, then the phase of immune escape is reached, eventually leading to the clinical manifestation of the disease. These phases together describe the theory of cancer *immunoediting*, which is a dynamic process that consists of *immunosurveillance* (the power of the innate and adaptive immune system to eradicate cancerous growth) and progression of the tumor.

A great deal of evidence proves that neoplastic lesions (rapid division of cells that form benign or malignant tumors) are under immunosurveillance, which is the monitoring process by which cells of the immune system (such as natural killer cells, cytotoxic T-cells, or macrophages) detect and destroy premalignant or cancerous cells in the body. Early proof of this was noted by pathologists who recognized that many patient tumors were densely infiltrated by innate and adaptive immune cells. The latest studies demonstrate that these immune cells are mounting an antitumor response and that tumors develop mechanisms to combat an immune response.

Why can cancerous cells escape immune surveillance? Clearly, the immune system's surveillance of rogue cells plays a large part in the suppression of tumor escape, but for a variety of reasons cancers are still able to progress. Mechanisms of avoiding immune recognition are now being explored as new therapies.

CONCLUSION

Antitumor immunity is a key component in preventing reoccurrence and preventing breast cancer from developing. The tumor suppresses and evades the immune response for several reasons, some of which will be explored further in Part 2 of this text. The role of inflammation in breast tumor initiation and progression is also a major factor in breast cancer development, cancer spread, and whether or not you will have a reoccurrence. (See Chapter 9, "Looking Forward," on page 264.) Fortunately, new immunotherapeutic and immunoengineering strategies are emerging as a promising approach for the discovery and design of immune system-based strategies for breast cancer treatment.

In addition, a weakened immune system is one of the major possible side effects of chemotherapy and radiation that is not commonly discussed by oncology. It is, however, one of the most important systems that should be examined to help prevent a reoccurrence as well as to help avert the development of breast cancer. Chapter 8 of this book ("Strengthening Your Immune System") will review in detail your immune system, how it functions, as well as therapies that you can implement to strengthen this very important function in your body.

PART 2

Unchangeable and Controllable Risk Factors

3

Unchangeable Risk Factors for Breast Cancer

A risk factor is anything that increases your chances of getting a disease, such as breast cancer. But having one or more risk factors does not mean that you are sure to get the disease. There are some risk factors that you can work on changing; however, some are unchangeable. Non-modifiable risk factors for breast cancer are ones that are not changeable. In other words, they are not under your control, such as age, gender, and family history (inheriting certain gene changes). Does that mean, if you have a number of these risk factors, that you are going to get breast cancer? The answer is no. However, what it does mean is that the odds of you getting breast cancer is higher than those who have fewer risk factors going against them.

By knowing what these risk factors are, you have an opportunity to stay one step ahead of such a diagnosis. From making sure you have a mammogram every year to having a mastectomy for those who are at the highest risk, you can make the call. As long as you recognize the risks, you have that power. So, to take the first step, in this chapter we will focus on the non-modifiable risk factors for breast cancer. It is essential to understand these issues so that you will more easily be able to understand how diligent you may want to be concerning your own situation.

AGE

Your risk of developing breast cancer increases as you get older. Currently, about 80 percent of patients with breast cancer are individuals aged greater than 50, while at the same time more than 40 percent are those more than 65 years old. The risk of developing breast cancer is 1.5 percent at age 40, 3 percent at age 50, and more than 4 percent at age 70. As people age, abnormal changes in their cells are more likely to occur, and their exposure to potential carcinogens results in an increase in the development of cancer over time.

In 2016, approximately 99.3 percent and 71.2 percent of all breast cancer-associated deaths in America were reported in women over the age of 40 and 60, respectively. Therefore, it is necessary to have a mammography screening ahead of time in women ages 40 and older.

The exception is a subtype of cancer, which is triple-negative breast cancer that is aggressive and resistant to treatment. It is most commonly diagnosed in individuals under the age of 40.

DENSE BREASTS

Breast density is a known risk factor for breast cancer, with studies suggesting a four- to sixfold increase in risk for women with highly dense breast tissue. These studies have made density one of the strongest known breast cancer risk factors. It is important to understand that the density of breast tissue remains inconsistent throughout a woman's lifetime. Greater density of the breasts is commonly observed in females of younger age and lower body mass index (BMI), women who are pregnant or breastfeeding, as well as during the intake of both natural and synthetic hormone replacement therapy. Generally, the greater breast tissue density correlates with the greater breast cancer risk; this trend is observed both in premenopausal and postmenopausal females.

It has been proposed that screening of breast tissue density could be a promising, non-invasive, and quick method for women who are at increased risk of cancer. Recently, new legislation in several states requiring breast density notification in all mammogram reports has increased awareness of breast density. Estimates indicate that up to 50 percent of women undergoing mammography will have high breast density. Thus, with increased attention and high prevalence of increased breast density, it is crucial that primary care clinicians and patients understand the implications of dense breasts. It is paramount that women discuss with their healthcare provider the possible need for supplemental screening options as part of a larger framework for the evaluation of breast tissue, in order to decrease a person's risk of developing breast cancer if they have dense breasts.

EARLY ONSET OF MENSTRUAL CYCLES (MENARCHE) AND BREAST DEVELOPMENT (THELARCHE)

A woman has an increased risk of breast cancer if her lifelong estrogen exposure is increased due to an early *menarche*, a late menopause, and/or an absence of childbearing.

For decades, it was presumed that the number of years of having your period, and consequently being exposed to estrogen longer, increased a woman's risk of developing breast cancer. However, recent epidemiological data have shown that early menstruation has a more significant effect on cancer risk than late menopause. Thus, rather than the overall years that you have had a menstrual cycle and were exposed to estrogen, it was found that this length of time plays less of a role than the timing of when her cycle started and when she was first exposed to hormones. Consequently, the older a woman is when her period begins, which is the first occurrence of menstruation, the lower her risk of getting breast cancer.

Several studies have now shown that starting your cycles prior to 11 years of age increases your risk of breast cancer, while a later age at menarche, such as 14 years, reduces the risk. Specifically, Dr. Andrea Sisti and colleagues showed that the relative risk of breast cancer was increased by five percent for each year younger at a woman's first menstrual cycle. In another trial, the Collaborative Group on Hormonal Factors in Breast Cancer (CGHFBC) reported up to an 18 percent reduction in risk in girls experiencing a late menarche (at 13 or older), compared to those who began cycling at 11. Also, there is a 23 percent increased risk of developing breast cancer associated with breast development prior to ten years of age. Furthermore, early menarche is a risk factor for breast cancer in women with and without a family history of breast cancer.

Likewise, while the age at menarche has been stable over the past half-century, the age at which breasts develop has continued to decrease. Causes of this rapid decline in age in breast development are not known. However, increasing rates of childhood obesity and changes in environmental factors, such as exposure to endocrine-disrupting chemicals and psychosocial stressors, are suggested to contribute to this trend. Recently, earlier breast development and a longer time between breast development and menarche were also shown to be associated with increased breast cancer risk.

In fact, the timing of breast development (*thelarche*) may be more biologically relevant to breast cancer risk than the timing of menarche. An early breast development can result in a longer period of exposure to estrogen, the hormone associated with breast cancer growth. In a recent study, earlier thelarche and the longer time period between breast development and menarche were independently associated with a 20 to 30 percent increased risk of breast cancer.

In that study, earlier age at reaching adult height was also associated with increased breast cancer risk. In addition, having both early breast development and early menarche was associated with an even greater increase in risk than experiencing only one of these pubertal events at an early age. Moreover, the age at menarche is inversely associated with both hormone receptor-positive and hormone receptor-negative disease.

Besides the time of estrogen exposure, examining other risk factors associated with earlier puberty may increase breast cancer risk by increasing the time that breast cells are in a highly proliferative, undifferentiated state that leaves them more susceptible to carcinogenesis (cancer development). Consequently, the time between breast development and menarche is considered biologically relevant to breast cancer risk since the majority of ductal development occurs during this timeframe. Likewise, puberty is a period of rapid breast development and a window of susceptibility for breast cancer risk, as the developing tissue may be particularly vulnerable to carcinogenesis. Lastly, early age at menarche is also associated with a worse tumor grade and lymph node involvement along with possibly an overall poorer prognosis.

The bottom line to keep in mind is this—the earlier the age that menarche starts, and breast development begins, the greater the risk is for breast cancer to develop.

OLDER AGE AT MENOPAUSE

Starting menopause after age 55 increases a woman's risk of breast cancer. The reverse is also true. Early menopause, despite whether natural or brought on through a surgical procedure, lowers the breast cancer risk.

Women with natural menopause at age 55 or older had twice the breast cancer risk experienced by those whose menopause occurred before age 45. The relative risk of breast cancer associated with late natural menopause was greatest after age 70. Each one-year delay in menopause increases the risk of breast cancer by three percent. The timing of menopause has been shown to significantly affect breast cancer risk.

Large-scale case-control studies and meta-analyses have now consistently shown that a younger age at menopause decreases ER+ breast cancer risk. Each year older at menopause increases the risk by 2.9 to 4 percent. However, it should also be kept in mind that women with an earlier age at menopause, and ER+ and/or PR+ stage I-III breast cancer, were more likely to develop metastatic breast cancer.

WOMEN WHO HAVE NOT GIVEN BIRTH (NULLIPARITY)

Nulliparity refers to a state in which a woman has not given birth to a child, although it doesn't necessarily mean she has never carried a pregnancy. The word "parity" refers to the number of times a woman has given births after 20 weeks of gestation. This includes someone who has had a miscarriage, still-birth, or an elective abortion.

Numerous studies confirmed that there is a strict relationship between exposure to endogenous hormones—estrogen and progesterone, in particular—and excessive risk of breast cancer in females. Consequently, if a woman has not had children, she is at an increased risk of developing breast cancer. Conversely, if she has had children, it provides lifelong protection against breast cancer by up to 50 percent. The protection provided by parity is restricted to hormone receptor positive tumors (ER+, PR+) only. In addition, protection was observed in studies at approximately 34 weeks and not confirmed for pregnancies lasting for less than 33 weeks.

As women around the world in industrialized countries are tending to have children at a later age or choosing not to have children, this issue should be discussed between the woman and her healthcare provider so that the woman can always make an informed decision that is best for her.

PERSONAL AND FAMILY HISTORY OF BREAST CANCER

Nearly a quarter of all breast cancer cases are related to family history. Women whose first-degree relative, their mother or sister, had breast cancer are more prone to this disease. A family history of breast cancer constitutes a major factor significantly associated with an increased risk of breast cancer. Approximately 13 to 19 percent of women diagnosed with breast cancer report a first-degree relative affected by the same condition. Furthermore, a study revealed that even with adjustment for breast density, a history of breast cancer in both first- and second-degree relatives is more strongly associated with breast cancer than simple first-degree family history.

Besides, the risk of breast cancer significantly increases with an increasing number of first-degree relatives affected. The risk might be even higher when the affected relatives are under 50 years old. In fact, the incidence rate of breast cancer is significantly higher in all women with a family history despite the age. This association is driven by heritable changes as well as environmental factors acting as potential triggers.

A study of over 113,000 women in the UK demonstrated that women with one first-degree relative with breast cancer have a 1.75-fold higher risk of developing this disease than women without any affected relatives. Moreover, the risk becomes 2.5-fold or higher in women with two or more first-degree relatives with breast cancer. The inherited susceptibility to breast cancer is partially attributed to the mutations of breast cancer related genes, such as *BRCA1* and *BRCA2*.

Furthermore, a history of any other non-cancerous alternations in breasts, such as atypical hyperplasia, carcinoma *in situ*, or many other proliferative or non-proliferative lesions, also increases the risk significantly. Atypical hyperplasia of the breast is the development of precancerous cells in the breast. Atypical hyperplasia causes a buildup of cells in the breast tissue. When viewed with a microscope, the cells look different from typical breast cells. Atypical hyperplasia of the breast isn't breast cancer. But it's a sign that you have an increased risk of breast cancer in the future.

In addition, the histological classification of benign lesions and a family history of breast cancer are two factors that are strongly associated with breast cancer risk.

Lastly, a personal history of breast cancer is associated with a greater risk of renewed cancerous lesions within the breasts.

GENETIC MUTATIONS

As we have explained, heredity plays an important role in breast cancer, but less than 30 percent of patients with a family history of breast cancer have specific predisposing genes. The most common cause of hereditary breast cancer is the genetic mutation in the BRCA1 and BRCA2 genes. The *BRCA* is short for BReast CAncer 1 and 2 genes. Other gene mutations can also lead to inherited breast cancer, such as *PTEN* (Phosphatase and TENsin homolog), *TP53* (Tumor Protein 53), *CDH1* (CaDHerin-1), and *STK11* (Serine/Threonine Kinase-11). They are primarily linked to the increased risk of breast carcinogenesis. The mutations within the above-mentioned genes are mainly inherited in an autosomal dominant manner. Autosomal means that the gene in question is located on one of the numbered, or non-sex, chromosomes. Dominant means that a single copy of the mutated gene (from one parent) is enough to cause the disorder. However, sporadic mutations are also commonly reported which are mutations that are not inherited.

BRCA1

By far the most prevalent and researched genes, *BRCA1* (located on chromosome 17) and *BRCA2* (located on chromosome 13) are characterized by a high penetrance. The penetrance in this case describes how likely a woman who carries any mutation of the BRCA1 or BRCA2 will develop breast cancer during her lifetime; some will, and some will not. They both encode tumor suppressor proteins. BRCA1 deficiency leads to the dysregulation of cell cycle checkpoint (mechanisms that monitor the events of the cell cycle), abnormal centrosome (plays an important role in cellular function and cell division) duplication, genetic instability, and, eventually, apoptosis.

BRCA2

The BRCA2 protein regulates recombinational repair in DNA double-strand breaks by interacting with the RAD51 gene and the DMC1 gene. BRCA2-associated breast cancers are more likely to be high-grade invasive ductal carcinomas. Women who carry a deleterious mutation (genetic alteration that increases a woman's predisposition) in BRCA1 or BRCA2 have high lifetime risks of breast and ovarian cancers. However, the influence of a family history of these cancers on these risks in women with BRCA mutations is unclear. A medical trial examined the 10-year cumulative risks of developing breast cancer as 18.1 percent for women with a BRCA1 mutation and 15.2 percent for women with a BRCA2 mutation. Among women with a BRCA1 mutation, the risk of breast cancer increased by 1.2-fold for each first-degree relative with breast cancer before age 50 years and the risk of ovarian cancer increased by 1.6-fold for each first- or second-degree relative with ovarian cancer. Among women with a BRCA2 mutation, the risk of breast cancer increased by 1.7-fold for each first-degree relative younger than 50 years with breast cancer.

In other words, about 20 to 25 percent of hereditary breast cancers and five to ten percent of all breast cancers are caused by BRCA1/2 mutations. Identification of the other more minor genes is not performed routinely in the clinical setting.

c-Myc

This gene is a multifunctional transcription factor (Myc protein) that directs the expression of genes required for rapid cell division while at the same time inhibiting expression of genes with antiproliferative functions. Some of the Myc-regulated genes such as *MTA1*, *hTERT*, and *PEG10* play vital roles in breast cancer initiation and if the disease progresses. The overexpression of c-Myc is mostly observed in the high-grade, invasive stage of breast carcinomas, while no c-Myc increase is detected in the benign (non-cancerous) tissues.

Epidermal Growth Factor Receptor (EGFR)

The Epidermal Growth Factor Receptor gene, EGFR, also known as *c-erbB-1* or *Her1* in humans, is a protein on cells that helps them grow. EGFR plays a role in cell-signaling pathways that control cells' division and survival. Over-expression of EGFR is found in more than 30 percent of cases of inflammatory breast cancer (IBC), a very aggressive subtype of breast cancer. Patients with *EGFR*-positive (a mutation in the gene that makes it grow too much) IBC have a poorer prognosis than those with *EGFR*-negative tumors. More than half of triple-negative breast cancer (TNBC) cases, characterized by the absence of estrogen receptor (ER), progesterone receptor (PR) expression and HER2 amplification, also have EGFR overexpression.

HER2

An HER2 positive breast cancer is a breast cancer that tests positive for the Human Epidermal growth factor Receptor 2 protein, also known as *c-erbB-2*. It is an important oncogene (a structurally and functionally heterogeneous group of genes) in breast cancer. This protein promotes the quick growth of cancer cells. Overexpression of HER2, when the cancer cells have extra copies of the gene that makes the protein, is detected in about 20 percent of primary breast cancers. Experts consider HER2 positive breast cancer to be more aggressive than some other breast cancers.

Ras

The *Ras* gene is short for "Rat Sarcoma Virus," and its three main members in the Ras gene family—*H-ras*, *K-ras*, and *N-ras*—encode proteins that play a crucial role in cell signaling that control cell growth and cell death. H-ras over-expression is detected in both primary and advanced breast cancer individuals where a poor prognosis is indicated.

Identifying a Potential Genetic Risk

Is there something you can do to learn if you are at risk because of your genetic make-up? As it turns out, breast surgeons routinely give genetic tests to iden-tify the type of cancer they are dealing with. However, if your family has a history of breast cancer, you might check with a doctor specializing in breast health to have a genetic test taken. A number of health insurance policies cover the cost of these tests. If this is a consideration, check with your health insurance company to learn if they do.

Once the results of the test are back, the names of the genes that have been identified should be listed. Since it's likely you aren't an expert on the subject of genetics, don't be afraid to ask your doctor what the results mean. The more informed you are, the better decisions you can make.

How Race and Ethnicity Affects Your Breast Cancer Risk

Your race or ethnicity does matter when considering your risk of developing breast cancer and the type of breast cancer. The mechanisms are not understood. Commonly, the incidence of breast cancer remains the highest among white non-Hispanic women. Conversely, the mortality rate due to this cancer is much higher among Black women and also has the lowest survival rates. Some researchers suggest that the mortality rate is higher in the Black population due to a decrease in availability of affordable health care.

Black women are twice as probable to get triple-negative breast cancer, an aggressive form that spreads quickly and is more difficult to treat. The data shows that Black women under the age of 35 have breast cancer rates that are two times above that of white women at an identical age.

White women, in contrast, possess the second highest mortality rate, followed by Native American, Hispanic, and Asian/Pacific Islander women.

DES DAUGHTERS

Diethylstilbestrol, commonly referred to as DES, is a synthetic form of the female hormone estrogen. It was prescribed as a medication to pregnant women between 1940 and 1971 to prevent miscarriage, premature labor, and related complications of pregnancy. The use of DES declined after studies in the 1950s showed that it was not effective in preventing these issues. However, in spite of the studies, it continued to be used to prevent lactation, for emergency contraception, and to treat menopause. With the use of this synthetic form of estrogen, the question was raised: Do the daughters of those mothers who used DES have a greater chance of getting breast cancer?

To answer this question, several studies were undertaken. In a 2006 study done in the United States, it was suggested that breast cancer risk was not increased in DES daughters overall—but that after age 40, DES daughters have approximately twice the risk of breast cancer as women not exposed at the same age and with similar risk factors. In addition, a 2011 study also found that a large group of DES daughters had nearly twice the risk of developing breast cancer at 40 years or older as unexposed women. There are, however, treatments that are available for DES daughters to consider, helping to mitigate the risk of developing breast cancer.

As a thought, for DES daughters who have families, there is not a lot of research on the effects of DES on the children of DES daughters and sons, so it may be a good idea to let them know about their exposure and to encourage them to have annual breast examination to know about the risks of exposure to DES.

Effects of DES on DES Daughters

DES has been linked with several health effects, some of which are related to an increase in breast cancer development. These include:

- Abnormal estrogen production and receptor function
- Abnormal glucose tolerance, which increases your risk of diabetes
- Abnormal progesterone production and receptor function
- Changes in levels of estradiol (E2 estrogen)
- Elevated levels of prolactin
- Higher rates of benign and malignant breast tumors
- Higher rates of uterine tumors, both benign and malignant
- Immune system dysfunction (changes in the T-helper and natural killer cells)
- Increased frequency of ovarian cysts and abnormal follicles
- Increased rates of endometriosis
- Increased risk of obesity
- Variations in concentrations of FSH (follicle-stimulating hormone)

Treatments for DES Daughters

While DES daughters have no control over their exposure to DES, there are some things they can do throughout life to protect their health.

- Conduct a breast self-exam at least once a month.
- Discuss DES with family and especially children. There is not a lot of research on the effects of DES on the children of DES daughters and sons, but it is a good idea for them to know about the risks of exposure to DES.
- Schedule regular mammograms and clinical breast examinations. Studies have shown that DES daughters over the age of forty have a greater risk of breast cancer, but younger DES daughters should get checked routinely as well.

- Schedule regular visits to the gynecologist, including Pap smears and pelvic exams. Special precautions during examinations may need to be taken with DES daughters.

- Seek infertility counseling, since many DES daughters have difficulty becoming pregnant.

- Treat all pregnancies as if they are high-risk.

IF YOU ARE AT HIGH RISK

If you have some of these risk factors, it is important that you conduct a breast self-examination at least once a month. It is equally important that you see your healthcare provider for yearly breast examinations. Furthermore, discuss your concern with your doctor and schedule a regular mammogram and/or thermogram.

CONCLUSION

Although some risk factors for breast cancer are controllable, there are those that are fixed, ones you cannot change, such as those described in this chapter. For some, managing the risk of developing breast cancer can be overwhelming, especially if you have a genetic susceptibility to breast cancer. However, there are things you can do, such as regular screening. Screening won't reduce the risks, but it can improve the chances of a good outcome if you are diagnosed early enough. Due to continuing research, scientists are learning more about breast cancer risk and risk factors. It is this knowledge that helps to upgrade and personalize detection and screening, reduce diagnoses, and, hopefully, prevent the disease entirely one day.

Now the question can be asked: Is there anything I can do to reduce my odds of getting breast cancer? The answer, in this case, is yes! Over the next few chapters, we will take a look at what these controllable risk factors are, and what we can do to protect ourselves.

4

Controllable Lifestyle and Nutrition Factors

n a recent report, the World Cancer Research Fund International (WCRF)/ American Institute for Cancer Research (AICR) estimated that, encompassing the thirteen most common cancers, 29 percent of cases could have been prevented by a healthy lifestyle. This includes breast cancer. Lifestyle and nutrition factors are major controllable risk factors for this disease. Knowing these factors and taking proactive steps to lower your chances of developing breast cancer, or getting the disease again, are key to you taking control of your own health care.

As you will learn, the information in this chapter can play an important role in lowering your odds of developing this disease. Most of these suggested changes are relatively easy to incorporate into your everyday life. Yes, it may take some willpower, but as the research shows, it will be well worth the effort.

ALCOHOL CONSUMPTION

You may not think about it this way, but alcohol is liquid sugar. Studies have shown a consistently direct association between alcohol intake and the risk of developing breast cancer. Moreover, several studies showed that alcohol consumption increased the risk of breast cancer; in particular, ER-positive tumors in postmenopausal women. In addition, a recent study showed a positive association between alcohol consumption and *endogenous* (produced inside the body) estrogen levels and mammographic density in premenopausal women.

A major trial revealed that drinking even small amounts of alcohol is linked to an increased risk of breast cancer in women. To be specific, one study revealed that a four percent risk of developing breast cancer is present at intakes of up to one alcoholic drink a day. Heavy alcohol consumption, defined as three or more drinks per day, is associated with an increased risk of 40 to 50 percent. This translates into about 5 percent of breast cancer in Northern Europe and North America that is due to heavy alcohol intake. The conclusion of this study was that women should not exceed one drink a day, and women at elevated risk for breast cancer should avoid alcohol altogether or consume alcohol only occasionally.

How does drinking alcohol increase your risk of developing breast cancer? Daily alcohol consumption increases serum estrogen levels, particularly estrone (E1) but also estradiol (E2) and other forms of estrogen. Overall, the *amount* of alcohol someone drinks over time—not the type of alcoholic beverage—seems to be the most important factor in raising cancer risk. It does not matter, therefore, if the alcohol is in the form of beer, wine, liquors (distilled spirits), or other drinks. Furthermore, alcohol interferes with estrogen pathways in other ways such as affecting estrogen receptors. Also, alcohol may increase the activity of estrogen-receptor signaling in breast tumors. Moreover, alcohol intake often results in excessive fat gain with higher BMI levels, which additionally increases the risk.

Other hypotheses include direct and indirect carcinogenic effects of alcohol metabolites and alcohol-related impaired nutrient intake. Consequently, mounting evidence suggests that antioxidant intake, such as folate, may reduce alcohol-associated breast cancer risk because it neutralizes reactive oxygen species, a second-stage product of alcohol metabolism. Therefore, diets lacking sufficient antioxidants intake may further elevate the risk of breast cancer among women consuming alcohol.

SUMMARY

Consequently, if you drink alcohol, then try not to drink more than one drink a day. If you have a strong family history of breast cancer—like I do—then you may want to consider not drinking any alcohol. Avoiding or cutting back on alcohol may be an important way for many women to lower their risk of breast cancer. Similarly, alcohol intake after breast cancer diagnosis is associated with an increased risk of reoccurrence.

CIGARETTE SMOKING

Most people understand that cigarette smoking is a risk factor for heart disease, stroke, chronic obstructive lung disease (COPD), diabetes, lung cancer, and memory loss. However, cigarette smoking is also a *controllable* lifestyle risk factor for breast cancer. It is amazing that, knowing all of this, one billion people in the world still smoke cigarettes—and smoking-related illness costs greater than $300 billion a year in the US alone. Nicotine (the active ingredient in tobacco) is highly addictive, resulting in sustained tobacco use.

The potential role of smoking in breast cancer risk has been the subject of over 100 publications and numerous scientific reviews, as well as lively debates. Tobacco smoke contains thousands of chemicals, many of which are known to be mammary carcinogens. Although not initially thought to be a tobacco-related cancer, evidence has been accumulating over the last several decades concerning the role of both active smoking and secondhand smoking as a cause of breast cancer. Human health evidence has been systematically evaluated, not only by several independent researchers but also by several expert agency panels. These agency panels include those of the US Surgeon General, the International Agency for Research on Cancer, and a coalition of Canadian health agencies. Although the assessments have varied over time, the most recent weight of the evidence has suggested a potentially causal role for active smoking and breast cancer, particularly for long-term heavy smoking and smoking initiation at an early age.

The role of secondhand smoking and breast cancer is less clear, although there have been some suggestions for an increased risk of premenopausal breast cancer. The European Prospective Investigation into Cancer and Nutrition conducted the largest cohort analysis on smoking and breast cancer to date. It found a higher risk of breast cancer diagnosis for women who were former and current smokers, and who were currently exposed to secondhand smoking, when compared with those who never smoked and those who were never exposed to secondhand smoke.

Most researchers agree that smoking may not only affect incidence rates but may *also* affect the survival of patients with previously established breast cancer. Moreover, the relative risk of breast cancer associated with smoking was greater for women with a family history of the disease. A longer smoking history, as well as smoking before the first full-term pregnancy, is an additional risk factor that is notable in females with a family history of breast cancer.

Several mechanisms have been proposed for the development of cigarette smoke-induced breast cancer. Various compounds in tobacco smoke, such as *polycyclic hydrocarbons* (chemicals found in coal, crude oil, and gasoline), *aromatic amines* (chemicals found in commercial hair dyes, diesel exhaust, and industrial plants), and *N-nitrosamines* (found in detergents and pesticides) may induce breast tumors. In addition, carcinogens found in tobacco are transported to the breast tissue, thus increasing the plausibility of mutations within oncogenes and suppressor genes (*p53*, in particular). *Oncogenes* are the main genes contributing to the changing of normal cells to cancer cells, while *tumor-suppressive genes* bar the development of cancer. As a result, both active and passive smoking contribute significantly to the induction of pro-carcinogenic events.

The active smoking evidence bolsters support for three studies, each of which reported a 65 percent increase in premenopausal breast cancer risk among smokers never exposed to secondhand smoke. In addition, prospective studies have generally found that smoking-related exposures were more consistently and strongly associated with ER+ than ER- breast cancer risk. Furthermore, a recent comparative study (Luo et al.) found a nine percent increased risk of breast cancer between former smokers and nonsmokers. This risk was even greater at 16 percent for current smokers. In support, yet another recent study showed that smoking 40 or more cigarettes per day had the strongest association with the risk of breast cancer.

Moreover, another trial found breast cancer to be associated with duration, intensity, cumulative exposure, and *latency* (the state of existing, but not yet developed or having manifested itself). These results strongly support the role of cigarette smoking as a cause of breast cancer and emphasize the importance of timing of this exposure. Consequently, the results from laboratory studies provide a compelling case for the role of cigarette smoke-mediated breast cancer development and progression.

The most notable starting point for the basis of these studies was to discover if cigarette smoke components reach the breast tissue. Components of cigarette smoke have been found in the nipple aspirate of female smokers. In addition, the presence of smoking-related DNA adducts in epithelial cells of breast milk demonstrates that cigarette components *can* access breast tissue. Likewise, the formation of DNA adducts has been proven to be a widespread mechanism for tumor development as a result of cigarette smoking. A DNA adduct is a segment of DNA bound to a cancer-causing chemical. Smoking-induced mechanisms underlying tumor progression and metastasis have also been reported.

Lastly, important studies have identified increased motility and epithelial-mesenchymal transition (EMT) in breast tumor cells exposed to cigarette smoke. The epithelial-mesenchymal transition (EMT) is a process by which *epithelial cells* (cells lining the internal and external surfaces of the body) lose their cell polarity (asymmetry in molecular composition) and cell-cell adhesion, and gain migratory and invasive properties. Therefore, it is a key step in the *transdifferentiating* process (conversion of one differentiated cell type into another cell type) in solid cancer development.

If you have already been diagnosed with breast cancer, does cigarette smoking affect your survival rate? Several studies have investigated patients who have already developed breast cancer and their risk. Another study (Pierce et al) found that breast cancer patients who were former smokers with more than a "30-packs-a-year" history had a 37 percent increased risk of breast cancer reoccurrence and 54 percent increased risk of overall breast cancer mortality when compared with non-smoking patients. Moreover, the overall mortality from any cause increased by 60 percent for these heavy smokers.

HARMFUL CONTENTS OF TOBACCO SMOKE

Cigarette smoking has a negative effect on your health due to what is in tobacco smoke. It is not just nicotine. In his book *Never Smoke Again*, Grant Cooper, MD, lists the following as just a fraction of the harmful contents that are found in cigarette smoke, some of which are related to the development of cancer. For example, preliminary evidence suggests a potential relationship between levels of arsenic exposure and breast cancer risk.

- Acetone
- Arsenic
- Benzene
- Butadiene (a flammable hydrocarbon)
- Carbon monoxide

- Cyanide
- DDT (insecticide)
- Dieldrin (hazardous chemical used in insecticides)
- Formaldehyde

- Lead
- Naphthalene (used to make mothballs)
- Styrene (used to make Styrofoam)
- Vinyl chloride

■ NICOTINE ADDICTION

Nicotine, a highly addictive chemical, is both physically and psychologically habit-forming. Cigarette smoke is physically addictive (since habitual users come to crave the chemical components) and mentally addictive, given that users *knowingly* desire the effects of nicotine. Most people go through withdrawal symptoms when they try to quit smoking. You may experience some—but probably not *all*—of these if you are trying to quit smoking:

- Anxiety
- Constipation
- Cough
- Cravings
- Depression

- Difficulty concentrating
- Dizziness
- Dry mouth
- Fatigue
- Headache

- Hunger
- Insomnia
- Irritability
- Postnasal drip
- Sore throat

TREATMENTS TO HELP YOU BREAK THE HABIT

Several treatments are available to help you quit smoking by getting you past your craving for nicotine. These include both conventional therapies—including behavioral support—and Personalized Medicine therapies.

CONVENTIONAL THERAPIES

Since the development of *nicotine replacement therapy* (NRT) in 1978, treatment options have continued to evolve and expand to aid individuals in smoking cessation. Despite this, currently available treatments remain insufficient, with less than 25 percent of smokers remaining abstinent one year after treatment. The two main approaches to assist cessation are pharmacotherapy and behavioral support.

Pharmacotherapy

Pharmacotherapy for smoking cessation aims primarily to reduce the intensity of urges to smoke and/or ameliorate the aversive symptoms. These are all prescription medications and may cause significant side effects in some individuals. They also may interact with other medications. Make sure that you have a long discussion concerning the "pros" and "cons" of each of these medications before starting drug therapy.

Behavioral Support

Behavioral support aims to boost motivation to resist the urge to smoke and develop a person's capacity to employ their plans to avoid smoking. These interventions usually last only a few months. The goal is that during these months, the strength of the associative learning between smoking and reward diminishes and most symptoms of withdrawal remit. After these few months, most smokers should have overcome their addiction and should be able to remain off cigarettes. Hypnosis has also been shown to be effective for some individuals. Furthermore, a good exercise program may be helpful since it serves as both a distraction as well as a form of meditation. Exercise also has a positive effect on mood. Studies have shown that a combination of both a behavioral and pharmacological approach is more effective in smoking cessation than either approach alone.

PERSONALIZED MEDICINE THERAPIES

Personalized Medicine therapies have also been shown to be beneficial for some patients, including:

- Novel therapies, such as *n-acetyl cysteine* (NAC), are displaying promising results. N-acetyl cysteine has antioxidant properties, both increasing glutathione and modulating glutamatergic, neurotropic, mitochondrial, and inflammatory pathways. It is well-tolerated, with a side effect profile that does not differ significantly from placebo in clinical trials when given orally at doses up to three grams a day, the exception being mild gastrointestinal side effects. NAC may also improve some of the physical harm caused by tobacco smoke exposure, including mucociliary transport, which is the self-clearing mechanism of the airways in the respiratory system. NAC also prevents oxidative damage to the lungs and other tissues.

- Studies have found that people who smoke, and those who are exposed to secondhand smoke, have reduced amounts of vitamin C in their bodies. Smokers should take an additional 2,000 mg of vitamin C a day.

- Tai chi, acupuncture, yoga, hypnotherapy, and mindfulness meditation have also been shown to be helpful.

SUMMARY

In summary, it is reasonable to conclude that long-term cigarette smoking provides a clear risk for many disorders from lung cancer to heart disease, to cognitive decline. It is also associated with the development of breast cancer and worsening of the disease. Several cohort studies have shown that longer duration, increased amount, and the beginning age of smoking are associated with high risk of breast cancer. Consequently, tobacco smoking is among the leading preventable risk factors for various diseases including breast cancer. Fortunately, there are many treatments both conventional and from a Personalized Medicine approach to help you break the habit.

FIRST PREGNANCY AFTER THE AGE OF 30

Pregnancy is one factor that is known to influence the chances of a woman developing breast cancer. Women who become pregnant and have children at an early age have a decreased risk of developing breast cancer in later life.

The first full-term pregnancy at an early age (especially in the early twenties), along with a subsequently increasing number of births, are associated with a reduced risk of breast cancer. To be specific, protection was observed at approximately the 34th week of pregnancy—and not for women that terminated their pregnancy or miscarried *before* 34 weeks.

Also, from the numerous studies of breast cancer risk, there is a consensus that an early first birth and increasing number of full-term births are associated with a long-term reduction in risk. The older a mother is at the age of the first full-term birth, however, the less the protection that is instilled by the pregnancy. Additional births provide an extra ten percent reduction in risk. Moreover, the spacing between births can influence breast cancer risk as well.

Pregnancy causes extensive changes to the breasts, making breast cells less likely to multiply and less likely to develop tumors—which could explain the protective effect of pregnancy for women who are younger. After age 35, breast tissue is more likely to have accumulated cells carrying cancer-causing mutations, or clusters of abnormal cells with the potential to become cancerous. However, it was not known for many years how these cells were affected by a late-age first pregnancy.

Now, researchers at Baylor College of Medicine, the MD Anderson Cancer Center, and the University of Colorado in Denver report that the answer to this question lies in what is called the JAK-STAT5 signaling pathway. This pathway is a chain of interactions between proteins in a cell, and is involved in processes such as immunity, cell division, cell death, and tumor formation. JAK-STAT signaling in mammary glands (located within breasts) can promote cell division and reduce cell death (apoptosis) during pregnancy and puberty—and therefore, if excessively activated, cancer can form. High STAT3 activity plays a major role in this process, as it can provide a pathway for genes, such as BCL2 and c-Myc, to initiate the process of cell division.

Recent reports have identified that more women in Western cultures are remaining childless, or *delaying* childbearing, until after 35 years of age. Therefore, it is proposed that this decline in childbearing and increasing age at first full-term birth may be contributing to the rise in breast cancer incidence.

SUMMARY

If you have not yet had children and you are under the age of 30, this risk factor can become a modifiable one if you choose to have children at a younger age. The great news is that you will see in subsequent chapters that if you have had children at an older age or choose to have them later in life, there are still many modifiable risk factors that can positively affect your risk of developing breast cancer along with decreasing your risk of a reoccurrence.

BREASTFEEDING

If you breastfeed, it decreases your risk of developing breast cancer significantly. Furthermore, there is a seven percent reduction following each birth study. In fact, studies conducted in 30 countries have confirmed this information. Similarly, a 2013 review of 32 studies concluded that the risk of having breast cancer was 14 percent lower among women who have given birth to one or more children and had breastfed, compared to women who have had children and never breastfed. This protective effect was even greater for women who had breastfed for 12 months or longer in their lives, an astounding 28 percent lower risk of developing breast cancer.

In contrast to the protective effects of childbearing, the protection conferred by breastfeeding is not limited to ER+ breast cancer. In addition, the longer duration of the breastfeeding period also reduces the risk of both ER/PR-positive and -negative cancers. Hormone receptor-negative breast cancers, which are more common in younger women, generally have a poorer prognosis than other subtypes of breast cancer.

Breastfeeding not only reduces breast cancer risk but also confers other health benefits to the mother, including reduced risk for endometrial and ovarian cancers and reduced risk for chronic conditions that are also risk factors for cancer, such as hypertension (high blood pressure) and diabetes. Additionally, breastfeeding provides many benefits to the infant, including fewer episodes of infections and a lower risk of sudden infant death, diabetes, asthma, and childhood obesity. This protection is believed to be conferred into young adulthood.

Interestingly, a study estimated that existing global breastfeeding rates prevent almost 20,000 annual deaths from breast cancer and that an additional 20,000 could be prevented by increasing breastfeeding duration to 12 months per child in high-income countries such as the US, and to 2 years per child in low- and middle-income countries.

SUMMARY

Of course, breastfeeding is an individual choice. For those who choose to breastfeed for 12 months, studies have shown that there is a four percent reduction in the risk of breast cancer. Research has also indicated that the longer the duration of breastfeeding beyond the first year, the greater percentage of reduction is achieved. However. for some women, it is not an option based on many factors such as social norms, embarrassment, poor family and social support, lactation problems, and employment and childcare. There are still many other things, however, that you can do to decrease your risk.

ORAL CONTRACEPTIVE USE

Oral contraceptives (birth control pills) are hormone-containing medications that are taken by mouth to prevent pregnancy. They do so by inhibiting ovulation, and also by preventing sperm from penetrating through the cervix. By far, the most commonly prescribed type of oral contraceptive both in the US and worldwide contains synthetic versions of the natural female hormones estrogen and progesterone. This type of birth control pill is often called a *combined oral contraceptive*. Another type of oral contraceptive, sometimes called the "mini-pill," contains only *progestin*, which is a man-made (synthetic) version of progesterone.

An analysis of data from more than 150,000 women who participated in 54 epidemiologic studies showed that, overall, women who had ever used oral contraceptives had a seven percent increase in the relative risk of breast cancer compared with women who had *never* used oral contraceptives. Women who were currently using oral contraceptives had a 24 percent increase in risk that did not increase with the duration of use. Risk declined after use of oral contraceptives stopped, and no risk increase was evident by ten years after use had stopped.

In 2017, a large prospective Danish study reported breast cancer risks associated with more recent formulations of oral contraceptives. A *prospective study* is an experimental design that looks forward in time and observes events as they happen. Overall, women who were using or had recently stopped using oral combined hormone contraceptives had about a 20 percent increase in the risk of getting breast cancer compared with women who had never used oral contraceptives. The risk increase varies from 0 percent to 60 percent, depending on the specific type of oral combined hormone contraceptive. The risk of breast cancer also increased the longer oral contraceptives were used. Additionally, long-term use of contemporary oral contraceptives and current use for five years or more was associated with an increased breast cancer risk among women ages 20 to 44.

A very new study found that "the relative risk of being diagnosed with breast cancer was 20 percent to 30 percent higher among women who used or recently used birth control pills with a two-hormone combination, progestogen-only pills, or hormonal IUDs compared to women who did not."

SUMMARY

Overall, these studies have provided consistent evidence that the risk of developing breast cancer is increased in women who use oral contraceptives or IUDs (intrauterine devices) that contain synthetic hormones.

EXERCISE

What is exercise? There is an important distinction between physical activity and exercise. Physical activity is a general term that can be applied to any movement that engages the muscles, ranging from daily chores such as gardening, making beds, or vacuuming, to rigorous sports like tennis, running, or swimming, all of which raise the heart rate and build endurance. The term exercise, however, refers to planned, purposeful movement specifically intended to boost physical fitness. Running, walking, biking, swimming, sports, hot yoga, and dancing are all activities that require effort, expend energy, and help to work core muscle groups.

AEROBIC VS. ANAEROBIC EXERCISE

Exercise is divided into two main categories: *aerobic* and *anaerobic*. Aerobic exercise (which is also called cardiovascular exercise) includes any activity that is rhythmic, continuous, and prolonged, and therefore increases your heart rate and requires an additional intake of oxygen. Running, cycling, swimming, skating, aerobic dancing, climbing stairs, and jumping rope are all forms of aerobic exercise.

Anaerobic exercise, on the other hand, requires very little increase in oxygen, as it is typically shorter in duration and of higher intensity. Weightlifting, sprinting, jumping, rowing, doing push-ups, doing sit-ups, and serving volleyballs or tennis balls are all examples of anaerobic exercise. These activities are generally strenuous, involve quick bursts of energy, and result in muscle fatigue rather than a deficit in oxygen.

Although anaerobic exercise builds strength and lean muscle mass, aerobic exercise is what health organizations like the American College of Sports Medicine (ACSM) are generally referring to when they give their recommendations for physical activity. According to the ACSM, American Health Association, and the US Surgeon General, adults need about 30 minutes of moderately intense cardiovascular activity (aerobic exercise) four or five days a week, or 20 minutes of vigorous cardiovascular activity three times a week.

The wonderful news is that exercise decreases the risk of developing breast cancer. A study found that the lifestyle factor most strongly and consistently associated with both breast cancer incidence and risk of breast cancer reoccurrence is physical activity. Another study supports the concept that moderate recreational physical activity (about 3 to 4 hours walking per week) may reduce breast cancer incidence. In addition, women with early-stage breast cancer who increased or maintain their physical activity may have lower reoccurrence risk as well.

Physical activity is recommended to avoid excessive weight gain. For example, the beneficial effects on the risk of breast cancer could be achieved by walking half an hour per day. Three to five hours per week of moderate physical exercise should therefore be considered for optimizing the reduction of the risk of cancer. For most women, moderate to intense activity—such as heavy housework, brisk walking, or dancing—could provide an effective level of activity to reduce the risk of breast cancer. The recent findings reveal that even minimal amounts of daily exercise and a healthy diet reduced the risk of breast cancer, mitigated the side effects of cancer treatment, and stopped the reoccurrence of cancer in the survivors.

The American Cancer Society recommends getting 150 to 300 minutes (2½ to 5 hours) of moderate physical activity a week, or 75 to 100 minutes (about 1 to 2 hours) of vigorous activity. This amount of activity is linked to a decreased risk of cancer overall. Moderate activities include walking, mowing the lawn, and slow dancing. Vigorous activities include jogging, playing tennis, and swimming. It's not just intense exercise that's related to a decreased risk of breast cancer. Women who get activity equal to taking a brisk walk 30 minutes a day have about a three-percent lower risk of breast cancer than women who aren't active. Another study showed even better numbers. In fact, overall, women who get regular exercise have a ten- to twenty-percent lower risk of breast cancer risk than women who aren't active. This benefit is seen most clearly in postmenopausal women.

Why is exercise linked to a decrease in breast cancer risk? Exercise is linked to a decreased breast cancer risk for several reasons:

- Exercise can help with weight control. Women who are lean have a lower risk of breast cancer after menopause compared to heavy women.

- Being active may also decrease blood estrogen levels. Women with lower blood estrogen levels have a lower risk of breast cancer than women with higher levels.

- Exercise boosts the body's immune system so it can help kill or slow the growth of cancer cells.

- Exercise also lowers blood sugar and fasting insulin levels. High levels are associated with an increased risk of getting breast cancer.

- Exercise has been shown to lower cortisol (stress hormone) levels. Abnormal cortisol levels are also associated with a higher rate of breast cancer.

How about individuals who have or have *had* breast cancer? Does it really matter if they exercise? The impact of exercise has been consistently studied within distinct phases of breast cancer therapy, including pre-breast-cancer treatment (for example, rehabilitation), during-breast-cancer treatment, after-breast-cancer treatment into survivorship, and living with metastatic breast cancer. In each of these phases, evidence has shown that exercise participation is a safe, viable, and effective means of providing functional, fitness, psychosocial, and treatment-related benefits.

In addition, the findings of a cohort study suggest that even moderate physical activity was associated with a 60 percent lower risk of death among breast cancer survivors. In another trial, exercise corresponding to 2.5 hours or more of brisk weekly walking after breast cancer diagnosis may reduce mortality by up to 32 percent compared to low-level exercise. Participation in an exercise program may reduce mortality by 44 percent compared to non-participation. Exercise is so important that many cancer centers tailor their exercise program for patients undergoing breast cancer treatment as well as for treatment-related impairments. Interestingly, if you have had breast cancer, some studies show being active after a breast cancer diagnosis is linked to a lower risk of both breast cancer-specific mortality, death from breast cancer, and overall mortality and death from any cause (not necessarily breast cancer).

SUMMARY

The evidence shows that exercise is safe and provides benefits in quality of life and in muscular and aerobic fitness for people with cancer, both during and after treatment, and should be continued over an individual's lifetime. Exercise also helps prevent one of the *major* possible side effects of cancer therapy—bone loss. A regular exercise program may also help prevent a reoccurrence. If you have not had breast cancer, studies have shown that exercise helps *prevent* breast cancer along with many other disease processes.

DIET

There is growing evidence that a poor diet may be associated with a higher breast cancer risk. Conversely, good eating habits decrease your risk of developing breast cancer and progression. Studies have shown that eating cruciferous vegetables (broccoli, cauliflower, Brussels sprouts, cabbage, and kale) decreases your risk of developing breast cancer, since their consumption improves the breakdown of estrogen in your body into components that decrease your risk. In addition, medical trials have shown that high fiber intake also decreases your risk of developing breast cancer.

MEDITERRANEAN DIET

A *Mediterranean diet* (a diet high in omega-3 fatty acids and vegetables) has been associated with a decreased risk for many diseases, including breast cancer in both premenopausal and postmenopausal women. The protective effect of the Mediterranean diet against the risk of breast cancer is due primarily to the principal foods of this eating program. The main components of the Mediterranean diet, such as fruits and vegetables, olive oil, and fish have important antioxidants properties due to their high content of substances like polyphenols, flavonoids, carotenoids, and fibers, along with a favorable fatty acid profile. That, in turn, could reduce your risk of developing breast cancer. It may also modulate breast cancer risk by decreasing endogenous estrogens, increasing sex-hormone binding globulin levels, neutralizing free radicals, and preventing DNA damage, along with reducing oxidative stress.

One study found that women who consume olive oil have a 25 percent lower risk of developing breast cancer. Furthermore, the intake of dietary *lignans* (compounds found in plants) found in flaxseeds have been known to decrease breast cancer risk.

SUMMARY

The *Standard American Diet* is just what the acronym says it is: SAD. The modern Western diet contains too much fat, especially saturated fat, which is associated with an increase in mortality and a poor prognosis in individuals with breast cancer.

Choosing a healthy eating program, such as a Mediterranean diet, goes a long way in helping prevent breast cancer as well as stopping a reoccurrence.

HIGH-FRUCTOSE CORN SYRUP (HFCS)

High-fructose corn syrup (HFCS) is a commonly used sweetener added to most beverages and processed foods. Extracted from corn and turned into syrup, it contains fructose, glucose, and water—and it is much cheaper to produce and sell than other sweeteners. It is one of the major reasons why our Western diet has such high calorie counts. While the low concentrations of fructose found in honey, fruits, and vegetables do not appear harmful, consumption has increased drastically over the past few decades—paralleling the increase in obesity, especially since the introduction of HFCS into processed foods was commercialized.

The consumption of large amounts of dietary sugar, and fructose in particular, has been associated with an altered metabolic state, both throughout the body and in specific tissues. This altered metabolic state (which will be discussed further) has many profound effects and is associated with many diseases, including diabetes, cardiovascular disease, and cancer. Specific types of cancer, such as triple-negative breast cancer (TNBC), are both responsive to dietary factors, and are exceptionally difficult to treat. This illustrates the possibility for preventative care through dietary intervention for people that have both controllable and uncontrollable risk factors for breast cancer. To treat obesity, diabetes, and cancer, it is imperative to understand systemic and localized metabolic abnormalities that drive their progression. Studies have shown that the incorporation of high- fructose corn syrup into everyday living is a key component of these metabolic changes.

As the second largest sugar ingested in the human body, fructose is an important source of fuel in the diet, especially in our Western diet. Fructose constitutes more than 40 percent of sweetener consumption in Western countries, in which high-fructose corn syrup consumption increased by more than 1,000 percent between 1970 and 1990. In addition, fructose has the highest sweetness among all natural sugars, and its sweetness is about 1.8 times that of sucrose. Sucrose, a disaccharide, is a sugar composed of glucose and fructose subunits. It is produced naturally in plants and is the main constituent of white sugar. The advantage to food manufacturers is that the free monosaccharides in HFCS provide better flavor enhancement, stability, freshness, texture, color, pourability, and consistency in foods in comparison to sucrose. The numbers are startling!

In preceding decades, the average person in the United States has shifted from eating 16 to 20 grams of fructose to consuming 60 to 150 grams *every day*. That's equal to between 4 and 15 tablespoons—almost one cup—of sugar daily. Furthermore, the increase in fructose consumption occurred in parallel with the increase in obesity. Obesity, which is associated with the chronic overconsumption of fructose, is also one of the largest predictors of breast cancer development. (See page 211 for a further discussion of this controllable risk factor.)

Additionally, it is important to note that fructose is more easily metabolized than glucose, because it bypasses the rate-limiting enzyme of the glycolytic pathway (which involves enzymatic reactions that break down glucose) and its metabolism is not controlled by insulin. Recent studies have revealed a correlation between excessive fructose consumption and tumor genesis and progression. In fact, one study revealed that fructose can be specifically used by breast cancer cells as a substitute for glucose, and the high-fructose diet could therefore accelerate the progress of breast cancer.

In fact, the capacity of fructose to produce advanced glycation end products (AGEs)—meats, cheeses, fried eggs, butter, cream cheese, margarine, mayonnaise, oils, and nuts, for example—that are generated through non-enzymatic glycation (attachment of a sugar to a protein, lipid, or nucleic acid molecule) in tissues, thereby altering tissue functions, is ten times greater than that of glucose. The common feature of this altered metabolism is the increased glucose uptake and fermentation of glucose to lactate. This phenomenon is known as the *Warburg effect*. Expanding evidence has demonstrated that the Warburg effect enables multiple invasive behaviors in triple-negative breast cancer, including:

- **Proliferation** (the growth of cells)

- **Metastasis reoccurrence** (the spread of cancer cells to other parts of the body)

- **Immune escape** (preventing our immune-fighting cells from responding to cancerous cells, and other pathogens)

- **Multidrug resistance** (allows cancer cells and other microorganisms to become resistant to a wide range of drugs)

Furthermore, while fructose does not directly stimulate insulin release, glucose production is increased in the body. Through these mechanisms, eating a lot of high fructose over time can lead to insulin resistance, which itself is a controllable risk factor for the development of breast cancer.

SUMMARY

The consumption of fructose is known to create distinct metabolic profiles—that is, how internal systems respond to stimuli and threats, both systemically and in individual tissues. The unregulated breakdown of fructose can strongly influence hepatic (liver) and systemic metabolism of glucose and lipid. Over time, this can lead to the development of multiple diseases, including obesity, diabetes, hypertension, non-alcoholic fatty liver disease, heart disease, and cancer.

Cancer cells rewire their metabolism to promote growth, survival, proliferation, and long-term maintenance. The common feature of this altered metabolism is the increased glucose uptake and fermentation of glucose to lactate. This phenomenon is observed even in the presence of completely functioning mitochondria and, together, is known as the Warburg effect. Breast cancer, in the form of triple-negative breast cancer, has been tied directly to an intake of a large amount of high-fructose corn syrup.

SUGAR INTAKE

Foods with *sugars added* make for extra calories in your diet but contribute little *nutritional value*. Refined sugar is 99.4 percent to 99.7 percent pure calories. There are no vitamins, minerals, or proteins. It is just carbohydrates. The body needs chromium, manganese, cobalt, copper, zinc, and magnesium to digest sugar. These minerals have been stripped from the sugar during the refining process. Consequently, the body depletes its own mineral reserves to process the sugar.

Predominantly, people can recognize desserts and candy as having added sugar, but how about the less obvious sources? Foods that most people would believe to be "healthy" may surprisingly have a lot of added sugar in them. There are hidden sugars in food that many people are not aware of. Just because the labels claim the product is "whole grain" or "fortified with vitamins and minerals," such as breakfast cereals, doesn't mean there's no sugar. In addition, some ketchups are one-half sugar; peanut butter may have sugar added; and sugar may be added to hamburgers sold in restaurants to decrease shrinkage.

Many major researchers and authors have examined the relationship between cancer and high sugar intake. Studies have shown that people who consume more sugar have an increased risk of developing cancer, particularly breast cancer. Likewise, in older women, a strong correlation was found between breast cancer mortality and sugar consumption. Consequently, epidemiological studies have also shown that dietary sugar intake has a significant impact on the development of breast cancer. For example, a ten-year trial of 101,279 participants from the French NutriNet-Sante prospective cohort study suggested that sugars may represent a controllable risk factor for cancer prevention, particularly breast cancer.

Importantly, specific types of cancer like triple-negative breast cancer (TNBC) are both responsive to dietary factors and very difficult to treat. Therefore, preventative care through dietary changes in at-risk populations is a must. One study showed a link between increased dietary fructose (a fruit and vegetable-based sugar) consumption, development of metabolic disturbances, and increased incidence of triple-negative breast cancer. (See the previous section in this chapter on high-fructose corn syrup for a longer discussion on this important topic.)

Does sugar intake affect you if you have already had breast cancer? A study prospectively documented 1,071 deaths due to breast cancer and 2,532 all-cause deaths, over a mean of 11.5 years of follow-up. After adjusting for confounding variables (an unmeasured *third* variable that influences both the supposed cause and effect), greater post-diagnosis total sugar intake was associated with a greater risk of breast cancer-specific mortality. Moreover, greater post-diagnostic fructose intake was significantly associated with greater risk of breast cancer-specific mortality and all-cause mortality. Furthermore, high post-diagnostic intake of sucrose was associated with higher risk of breast cancer-specific and all-cause mortality. Increased post-diagnostic intake of carbohydrate from fruit juice was also significantly associated with higher risk of breast cancer-specific and all-cause mortality.

Not surprisingly, a high post-diagnostic intake of carbohydrates from vegetables was associated with reduced risk of mortality. In addition, a large-scale study shows that high fruit and vegetable consumption may be associated with better overall survival among breast cancer patients, while high fruit juice consumption may be associated with poorer prognoses.

One proposed mechanism for how sugar impacts cancer development involves inflammation. For example, the intake of refined grains is associated with an inflammatory response. Another mechanism that is suggested for the increased risk of breast cancer development with high sugar ingestion is a study suggesting that dietary sugar induces the enzyme lipoxygenases (LOXs) signaling to increase the risk of breast cancer development and spread, which also increases inflammation in the body. In yet another additional study, coauthor Lorenzo Cohen, a professor at MD Anderson Cancer Center, determined that it was specifically fructose—in table sugar and high-fructose corn syrup, and existing virtually *everywhere* within our modern culture's food system—that was responsible for facilitating lung metastasis.

THE MANY FORMS OF SUGAR

Sugar comes in many forms, some of which are not as easily recognizable:

- Agave syrup or nectar
- Barley malt
- Beet sugar
- Brown sugar
- Cane sugar
- Cane syrup
- Confectioners' sugar
- Crystalline fructose
- Date sugar
- Evaporated sugarcane
- Fructose
- Fruit juice or concentrate
- Galactose
- Glucose
- Granulated sugar
- High-fructose corn syrup (HFCS)
- Honey
- Invert sugar (a liquid sweetener made from table sugar and water)

- Lactose
- Liquid cane sugar or syrup
- Maltose (malt sugar)
- Maple syrup
- Molasses
- Powdered sugar
- Raw sugar
- Rice syrup
- Sugarcane syrup
- Table sugar (sucrose)
- Turbinado sugar
- Unrefined sugar
- White sugar

SUGAR SUBSTITUTES

Trying to minimize the sugar and calories in your diet? You may resort to artificial sweeteners or other sugar substitutes if you cannot have sugar. These sugar substitutes are food additives, and they are equivalent to the taste of sugar—however, they have less food energy. Artificial sweeteners and other sugar substitutes are found in a range of foods and beverages advertised as "sugar-free" or "diet," including soft drinks and baked goods. What are all these sugar substitutes found in foods, and what role do they play in your diet? Let's examine each of the sugar substitutes.

- *Aspartame.* Aspartame, a non-saccharide artificial sweetener, is 200 times sweeter than sugar. Once your body processes aspartame, a portion of it is broken down into methanol. Methanol is toxic in sizable amounts, yet smaller quantities may also be worrisome. Since 2014, aspartame has been identified as the predominant source of methanol in the American diet. Research has recognized a link between aspartame and a host of conditions and possible following side effects.

- *Sucralose.* Sucralose starts with a sugar molecule and has three of its components removed and replaced with chloride. It provides no calories because the body does not recognize it as a food. Sucralose does not raise blood sugar but is 2,000 times sweeter than sugar. As of the FDA's approval in 1998, studies have surfaced about sucralose's possible negative side effects. The risks of consuming large quantities of sucralose may include diabetes, cancer, weight gain, and gastric issues. In addition, it may increase the development of hypothyroidism, since chloride may replace iodine in the body when using a lot of sucralose. Iodine is needed for optimal thyroid function. It is also an antibacterial, anticancer, antiparasitic, antiviral, and mucolytic agent.

- *Honey.* Honey contains small amounts of vitamins and minerals and is 20 percent to 60 percent sweeter than sugar. The primary argument behind the negative effect of consuming too much honey is the excessive amount of fructose existing in honey. This high proportion of fructose in honey diminishes the ability of the small intestine to metabolize nutrients appropriately.

- *Saccharin.* Saccharin, one of the oldest artificial sweeteners, has been used for over 100 years. Limited research exists on the side effects of saccharin; however, a possible link may exist between consuming saccharin in substantial amounts and high blood sugar and alterations in gut bacteria.

- *Stevia.* Stevia is extracted from a leaf and has no known side effects. It does not raise glucose or insulin (the hormone that regulates blood sugar) levels in the body.

- *Sugar alcohols.* Sugar alcohols are naturally occurring sweet compounds found in fruits and vegetables. Supplements are made from the fiber of birth trees. Sugar alcohols include: xylitol, sorbitol, mannitol, and isomalt. They may decrease the incidence of dental cavities. They fight plaque buildup and neutralize plaque acids. Sugar alcohols also increase satiety. They have 40 percent less calories than sugar and have a minimal effect on blood sugar and insulin levels. The body produces up to 15 grams of xylitol per day from other food sources. Sugar alcohols are incompletely absorbed in the intestine and may have a laxative effect, especially if used in large quantities.

Other artificial sweeteners that are currently permitted in the United States and other countries include: acesulfame potassium; neotame and advantame, which are both similar to aspartame; and luo han guo fruit extract. Refined sugars (e.g., sucrose and fructose) were absent from the diet of most people until very recently in history, which correlates with the significant rise in breast cancer that has occurred over the last 50 years.

SUGAR ADDICTION

Overconsumption of sugar-rich foods or beverages is initially motivated by the pleasure of sweet taste and is often compared to drug addiction in medical studies. One medical trial revealed that intense sweetness can surpass cocaine reward, even in drug-sensitized and addicted individuals. Sugar has been shown to activate opiate receptors in the brain, which affects the reward center, leading to compulsive behavior even though the individual knows that eating too much sugar may cause weight gain and have other negative effects upon the body.

In addition, excessive sugar intake causes an increase in the release of *dopamine*, a neurotransmitter that gives a person the feeling of a "high" and makes an individual want to repeat the behavior. In other words, in both animal and human studies, substantial commonalities are exhibited between drugs of abuse and sugar—from the standpoint of brain neurochemistry, as well as behavior.

SUMMARY

Consequently, one of the best ways that you can decrease your risk of developing breast cancer, as well as prevent a reoccurrence, is to decrease your intake of sugar. This is not an easy habit for many people to break—myself included—but it *can* be done.

VITAMIN D

Vitamin D may be involved in controlling normal breast cell growth and may be able to stop breast cancer reoccurrence. Research proposes that women with decreased levels of vitamin D have a higher risk of breast cancer. Studies have shown that women with the highest levels of vitamin D in their blood had a 45 percent decrease in the risk of breast cancer, in comparison to women with the lowest levels of vitamin D in their blood.

One can also get vitamin D from food, but only in small doses. Vitamin D_3 comes from red meat and fish, while vitamin D_2 comes from plants. In these forms, vitamin D must be metabolized in the body in order to be used by the body, and boron may be needed for the conversion. Vitamin D receptors are in the bones, pancreas, intestine, kidneys, brain, spinal cord, reproductive organs, thymus, adrenal glands, pituitary gland, and thyroid gland. Since vitamin D is fat-soluble, it is stored in the body's fat cells and liver. It is amazing, but a study indicated that almost 75 percent of people in the United States are vitamin D-deficient.

FUNCTIONS OF VITAMIN D

- Vitamin D plays a vital role in helping to protect older adults from osteoporosis. However, vitamin D has other functions in the body as well, including the reduction of inflammation and the modulation of such processes as cell growth and immune function. Vitamin D plays a key role in the readjustment of the inflammation system by regulating the production of inflammatory cytokines—signaling molecules and immune cells. Vitamin D deficiency has been associated with the rise of chronic inflammatory diseases. Vitamin D aids in modulating gene transcription, the process by which a cell makes an RNA copy of a piece of DNA—and the prevention and treatment of insulin resistance.

- Vitamin D receptor genes operated by vitamin D play key roles in the mammary gland through regulation of calcium transport during lactation, hormone differentiation, and milk production. Research has been directed toward identifying vitamin D as a breast cancer risk factor to be targeted for cancer prevention. This is because circulating vitamin D levels (levels greater or equal to 55 ng/mL) may protect against breast cancer. Breast cancer chemoprevention drugs change the process by which normal cells become cancer cells. These drugs have high toxicities and are commonly not effective in the aggressive estrogen receptor-negative (ER-) breast cancers.

CAUSES OF VITAMIN D DEFICIENCY

The following may lead to vitamin D deficiency:

☐ Aging process

☐ Decreased fat absorption (due to short bowel syndrome, celiac sprue, inability of the intestines to absorb nutrients from food, or certain medications)

☐ Fat-blocking medications and over-the-counter fat blockers used for weight loss

☐ Decreased exposure to the sun

☐ Medications such as phenytoin, phenobarbital carbamazepine, prednisone, and others

☐ Sunscreen use

SYMPTOMS OF VITAMIN D DEFICIENCY

Low vitamin D levels may result in signs/symptoms such as:

☐ Bone disorders (rickets in children, or softening of the bones in adults)

☐ Cognitive decline

☐ Decreased calcium levels

☐ Decreased phosphate levels

☐ Increased risk of bone loss

☐ Muscle spasms

RECOMMENDED DAILY DOSAGE

Consult your healthcare provider, who will order blood tests before deciding how much vitamin D you should consume. The fact is that each of our bodies uses vitamin D at different rates. So, while one person needs only 50 IUs of D per day to function appropriately, another person needs 1,000 IU daily to have the right amount for their internal system. By looking at the results of your blood test, a physician can tell you if you need more or less of this vitamin.

To get enough vitamin D from the sun's rays, you should expose your face and arms for ten to fifteen minutes, at least three times a week, without sunscreen. The use of sunscreen decreases the absorption of vitamin D into the skin. If you are very fair and need to wear sunscreen, then you may need to intake additional vitamin D. Studies have shown that the preferred form of vitamin D with which to supplement is vitamin D_3.

Food Sources

Vitamin D can be found in the following foods:

- Butter
- Canned sardines
- Liver
- Salmon
- Shrimp
- Sunflower seeds
- Tuna

SIDE EFFECTS AND CONTRAINDICATIONS

The optimal blood level of vitamin D is 55 to 80 ng/mL (120 to 160 nmol/L). Some people may not be able to supplement to an optimal level of vitamin D since they may develop high calcium levels in the body. This is called *hypersensitivity syndrome*. Hypersensitivity syndrome is commonly seen in people suffering from hyperparathyroidism, cancer, and granulomatous diseases such as sarcoid (pulmonary disease), Crohn's disease, and tuberculosis (TB). A *granulomatous disease* is a genetic condition in which white blood cells are unable to destroy certain types of bacteria and fungi. Consequently, for dosages over 1,000 IU a day, it is best to consult with your healthcare provider. It is necessary to take calcium when taking vitamin D.

SIDE EFFECTS OF VITAMIN D TOXICITY

Vitamin D is stored in the body. Therefore, individuals can become toxic. The following are possible side effects of vitamin D toxicity:

☐ Anorexia   ☐ Heart arrhythmias

☐ Hypercalcemia (elevated calcium levels in the blood)

☐ Hypercalciuria (elevated calcium levels in the urine)

☐ Joint pains

☐ Muscle weakness

☐ Nausea

☐ Polyuria

☐ Weight loss

Several studies have shown that there was a significant association found between low-serum calcitriol (the major circulating form of vitamin D in the body) levels and the risk of breast cancer development. In these studies, the majority of patients suffering from breast cancer were vitamin D-deficient. Moreover, results from a case-control study support the protective effect of higher-serum concentration of calcitriol against breast cancer. Likewise, dietary but not total intake of vitamin D was associated with decreased risk of breast cancer.

Recently, extensive research on its extra-skeletal actions has linked vitamin D deficiency to an increased risk of infection, diabetes mellitus types 1 and 2, cardiovascular disease, obesity, asthma, inflammatory bowel disease, colon, breast, prostate and ovarian cancer, and some neurological diseases.

BREAST CANCER AND VITAMIN D

There are various mechanisms by which vitamin D influences the progressive path of cancer development. These include the role of vitamin D in the induction of apoptosis (death of cells), stimulation of cell differentiation (the biological process of a cell developing and acquiring a more specialized form and function), anti-inflammatory and antiproliferative (stops cell growth), inhibition of angiogenesis (development of new blood vessels), invasion, and metastasis (the development of secondary malignant growths at a distance from a primary site of cancer).

Moreover, vitamin D modulates the activity of signaling pathways. Particularly in healthy breast cells, calcitriol (the active form of vitamin D) helps to control inhibition of cell growth and differentiation through intervention with vitamin D receptors. Yet another study suggested that the interruption of any of the multiple steps in the transport, metabolism, or function of calcitriol could contribute to the development or progression of breast cancer. Furthermore, research proposes that women with low levels of vitamin D present a higher risk of breast cancer.

Medical trials have suggested a role for vitamin D in prevention of breast cancer. As vitamin D levels go up, the risk of breast cancer development, risk for breast cancer reoccurrence, and mortality in women with early-stage breast cancer declines. Supplementation with vitamin D can reduce the risk of breast cancer in women, since it can downregulate the expression of estrogen receptors and attenuate the synthesis and signal of these hormones.

The following explains how vitamin D works to help prevent breast cancer and its spread, as well as its reoccurrence:

- **Growth arrest and cell death.** Experimental, preclinical, and ecological studies have shown that calcitriol induces differentiation and cell death and stops cell proliferation and angiogenesis, the formation of new blood vessels in normal and malignant breast cells.

- **Inhibition of invasion and metastasis.** In some breast cancer cell lines, calcitriol increases the expression of *E-cadherin*, a protein that prevents invasion and metastasis as well as other factors that are important mediators of cancer invasion and spread.

- **Anti-inflammation.** Calcitriol has been shown to reduce the responsiveness of the COX-2, an enzyme that plays a critical role in the synthesis of prostaglandin in several human breast cancer cell lines. A high expression level of COX-2 in breast cancer has been shown to correlate with high grade, large tumor size, and poor prognosis.

- **Estrogen pathway inhibition.** Several studies have suggested that calcitriol can inhibit both the synthesis and the biological actions of estrogens, including reducing the responsiveness of estrogen receptor (ER)-alpha, the nuclear receptor that enables the actions of estrogen.

- **Sunlight exposure.** Trials concerning breast cancer and vitamin D have shown strong inverse associations between sunlight exposure and breast cancer incidence and mortality. In fact, a study by Garland and his associates of eighty-seven US counties reported strong correlations between lower sunlight exposure and age-adjusted breast cancer mortality rates, with the highest rates in the Northeast when compared with the Southwest. In addition, several studies have shown a better prognosis for breast cancer patients following diagnosis or treatment initiation in the summer or fall. This seasonal effect was thought to be the result of greater vitamin D during a period of higher sunlight exposure at the time of diagnosis.

SUMMARY

As you have seen, it is possible that vitamin D plays a role in controlling normal breast cell growth and has the capacity to stop the growth of cancer cells.

This protective effect is believed to be largely supported by the chemo-preventive actions of calcitriol, the bioactive form of vitamin D.

CONCLUSION

The wonderful truth is that there are many things that you can do that are lifestyle-oriented and nutritionally related to help prevent breast cancer—and to keep from getting the disease *again*. The amount of alcohol consumed, and whether you smoke cigarettes or not, are easily modifiable risk factors for most people. Whether you breastfeed, if and when you have children, and if you use oral contraceptives are also contributing factors. Exercise and diet, of course, play a major role. The ingestion of high-fructose corn syrup has now been linked to breast cancer, as has a high intake of sugar in general. Moreover, it does matter if your vitamin D level is optimal—meaning perfect—instead of low or even normal. As you have seen, if your levels are optimal, it decreases your risk of developing breast cancer and a reoccurrence. Low or normal levels are not as protective. Fortunately, all these factors are something that you can control yourself to improve your risk.

5

Controllable Environmental Risk Factors

Perhaps in the very distant past, there was a time when our environment did not pose a danger to our health. The air was clean and the only thing our ancestors needed to live on were byproducts of nature. However, with the many advancements in science coupled with our societies' industrial needs, things have greatly changed. Today, we are all exposed to numerous toxic hazards—from the air we breathe and plastic bags we use to wrap products, to the foods we eat. We seem to be surrounded by a growing number of environmental risk factors, all of which have been shown to increase the possibility of developing breast cancer.

How is that possible, you may ask? As explained in the previous chapters, our bodies are made of various internal systems that allow us to carry on our daily lives. These systems are all made up of chemicals—starting from our skin right down to our genes. When the systems work, we are healthy; when the systems begin to falter, however, we get sick. When outside chemicals begin to disrupt these systems, beginning with our genes, the problems begin. And while these environmental toxins were never designed to create these types of health issues, they unfortunately have been found to do just that. By learning what some of these environmental risk factors are, you should be better able to lower your chances of developing any number of environmentally related disorders, including breast cancer.

AIR POLLUTION

Higher levels of some airborne metals—specifically, mercury, cadmium, and lead—were associated with a higher risk of postmenopausal breast cancer, as one study found. Furthermore, radon gas, which occurs naturally in the environment, can break down into radioactive particles that can mix with air pollutants. Such pollutants include carbon monoxide, nitrogen dioxide, ground-level ozone, and particulate matter. Researchers found that exposure to these airborne radioactive particles was associated with a higher risk of estrogen receptor-negative breast cancer. Moreover, researchers found that higher levels of nitrogen dioxide (NO_2), which is a component of air pollution related to traffic, were associated with higher rates of breast cancer.

How do you know if you might be exposed to "normal" air pollutants? If you experience the following symptoms—continuing eye irritation, wheezing, coughing, shortness of breath, a scratchy throat, and chest tightening—then you are likely to be in a polluted air zone. To learn more about the air quality in your specific area, you can go to the AirNow website at www.airnow.gov. This service is operated by the US Environmental Protection Agency. By submitting your location, this government agency can provide you with real-time information about your air quality.

If you find that the area you live in is heavily polluted with bad air, consider moving to an area that has cleaner air.

DRINKING WATER

In 1998, a study suggested an association between breast cancer and *perchloroethylene* (PCE; also called tetrachloroethylene) exposure from public drinking water. Drinking water contaminated by wastewater is a potential source of exposure to mammary carcinogens and endocrine-disrupting compounds from commercial products and excreted natural and pharmaceutical hormones. This chemical comes from manufacturing plants, stain removers, fragrances, degreasing products, and adhesives. Over time, this chemical finds its way into the water sites, the soil, and various water sources.

These contaminants are believed to increase breast cancer risk. Cape Cod, Massachusetts, has a history of wastewater contamination in many, but not all, of its public water supplies; and the region has a history of higher breast cancer incidence that is unexplained by the population's age, in-migration, mammography use, or established breast cancer risk factors. A follow-up study confirmed those of the previous one and suggested that women with the highest PCE exposure levels have a small to moderate increased risk of developing breast cancer.

This can be a concern for many people. Be aware that activated carbon filters and reverse osmosis filters can remove PCE from the water in your home. However, keep in mind that boiling water will *not* get rid of PCE in water.

ENDOCRINE-DISRUPTING CHEMICALS (EDCs)

Endocrine disruptors or *endocrine-disrupting chemicals* (EDCs) are substances in the environment that can interfere with the actions of hormones in your body; in other words, the ability to interfere with the action or metabolism of androgens, thyroid hormones, and steroid hormones. There is evidence that these hormonally active chemicals play a role in increasing your risk of developing breast cancer.

Endocrine-disrupting compounds are substances that are found everywhere in everyday life, including pesticides, plasticizers, pharmaceutical agents, personal care products, and in food products and food packaging. Increasing epidemiological evidence suggests that EDCs may affect the development or progression of breast cancer and consequently lead to lifelong harmful health consequences, especially when exposure occurs during early life. Through several mechanisms, endocrine disruptors have been linked to several cancers, including those of the thyroid, breast, and prostate.

Most studies reviewed environmental EDCs exposure through biomarker measurements. These studies have shown that certain EDC exposures could potentially elevate the risk of breast cancer. Since many EDCs are highly persistent in the environment and *bioaccumulative* (when chemicals accumulate in living organisms), it is essential to assess the long-term impacts of EDC exposures. Also, since food is often a major route of exposure to EDCs, well-designed exposure assessments of potential EDCs in food and food packing are necessary. In addition, their potential link to breast cancer development needs to be carefully evaluated for subsequent EDC policymaking.

Humans can be exposed to EDCs through different routes: (1) direct ingestion of contaminated food from packaging materials or additives that are deliberately added in food processing to help maintain the quality and safety of food products; (2) drinking of contaminated water; and (3) breathing of air and/or skin contacting contaminated soil, cosmetics, personal care products, and others. Food is the major route of EDC exposure. It is worth noting that the choices of diet would affect the levels of exposure to EDCs in humans. For example, people who eat a lot of oily fish, meat, and dairy products would have higher exposure to the more persistent EDCs—such as DDT (dichloro-diphenyl-trichloroethane)—than those who eat more vegetables, as the lipophilic- persistent EDCs are bioaccumulated in the lipid fraction of these foods.

Is there anything you can do to avoid endocrine-disrupting chemicals? Yes, there is. To learn how to spot these EDC products, the Endocrine Society provides a useful website, www.endocrine.org/topics/edc/what-you-can-do, that provides information on how to identify these products and what you can do to help make a difference.

A Good Endocrine Disruptor

Resveratrol (RES). Resveratrol is one of the polyphenols abundant in grape skin. Resveratrol has many functions in the body as an anti-inflammatory, antioxidant, protector of endothelial function (controlling blood fluidity, platelet aggregation, and vascular tone), and as something that helps lower the risk of heart disease, to name a few. It has been shown to decrease the risk of developing breast cancer. Resveratrol is structurally similar to estradiol, an estrogen hormone, and has endocrine disrupting properties. Unlike other phytoestrogens, it binds to estrogen receptor beta with higher affinity than estrogen receptor alpha, which decreases your risk of developing breast cancer. Several animal studies have shown that resveratrol is protective against mammary *tumorigenesis* (the process of gaining malignant properties). There is also a case-controlled study, which reported that taking resveratrol decreased the risk of developing breast cancer.

PESTICIDES

Regarding relationships between breast cancer and environmental factors in humans (outside of diet), the most compelling data comes from the exposure of pesticides through farming, which is associated with increased breast cancer incidences.

- **DDT and DDE.** The two pesticides with the most research linking them to breast cancer are *dichlorodiphenyltrichloroethane* (more commonly known as DDT) and its metabolite, DDE (dichlorodiphenyldichloroethylene). DDE is formed when DDT breaks down after exposure to sunlight. These two pesticides have always attracted a lot of attention worldwide because they are highly persistent EDCs in the environment. They can accumulate along the food chain and therefore immediately be detected in breast milk and adipose tissues (body fat). Most countries have imposed bans on the use of DTT. Studies reported higher levels of DDT or DDE among women with breast cancer than among controls.

- **TCDD (or dioxin).** *Dioxin* is one of the most infamous organochlorines that are formed as a result of combustion and manufacturing chemicals. Individuals can be exposed to dioxins through ingestion of foods that are high in fat content, such as meat, poultry, milk, eggs, and their related byproducts. Dioxins are fat-soluble, very persistent, and accumulate in the fatty tissues. They are considered as EDCs on the basis that they exert their *estrogenic* (mimicking natural estrogen) or *anti-androgenic* (keeping male sex hormones from binding to proteins) effects by binding to the *aromatic hydrocarbon receptor* (AhR) and inducing *epigenetic alterations* (heritable changes). The long-term effects of occupational exposure to dioxins, particularly with regards to cancer mortality, were also examined in a follow-up 23 years after closure of a German pesticide plant.

An increase in breast cancer mortality was found among women workers exposed to herbicides and insecticides. Similar results were observed in US women who live close to incinerator plants for a long period of time, compared to those who have lived farther away.

SYNTHETIC CHEMICALS

Synthetic chemicals are man-made and are deliberately created to replicate naturally occurring chemicals to be used in the creation of various products like pesticides, plastics, medicines, and lots more. While they mimic the effects of their natural counterparts, these chemicals are cheaper and easier to produce. Unfortunately, many of them come with side effects.

- **Bisphenol A (BPA).** Bisphenol A is a synthetic chemical used in manufacturing polycarbonate plastics for food and beverage storage. BPAs are also released into the environment through manufacturing industries like synthetic polymer and thermal paper, toys, table wares, and medical devices. Inhalation exposure occurs through dust from vinyl flooring, carpet backing, and consumer products such as fragrances, dryer sheets, air fresheners, and sunscreens.

  Most studies have shown that bisphenol A increases inflammatory markers such as C-reactive protein and IL-6. BPA is a known endocrine disruptor, and it was considered as a relatively weak environmental estrogen because of its ability to bind either ER alpha and ER beta, or their capacity to activate ER-dependent transcription. ER is a transcription factor regulating gene expression events that result in cell division. BPA was shown to induce tumor aggressiveness in breast cancer patients, which may be associated with a poor prognosis in one study. Consequently, BPA is considered as a potential risk factor for breast cancer. Moreover, recent studies have shown that high levels of bisphenol A are related to breast, thyroid, colorectal, ovarian, endometrial, and prostate cancer.

- **Phthalates.** Phthalates are a large class of chemicals that are constantly detected in food through food packaging materials and food contact substances used during processing and storage. They make plastics soft and flexible. They are found in a wide variety of common products including plastics, such as cosmetics, pharmaceuticals, baby care products, and children's toys. Phthalates are also found in building materials, modeling clay, automobiles, cleaning materials, and insecticides. In addition, they can also enter the body through inhalation, medical injection procedures, and are also easily absorbed through the skin. Moreover, many wines and liquors, and even spices, are contaminated with phthalates resulting from leakage of chemicals from storage containers. Studies have suggested a positive association of phthalates with breast cancer risk.

- **Genistein.** Genistein is a naturally occurring phytoestrogen found in most soy products. Although it is a *polyphenol*—a compound found in flowering plants, fruits, and vegetables—genistein shares structural similarity with estradiol (E2) and has been shown to act in a similar way as an estrogen. Laboratory, animal, and human data has shown that genistein can signal through both ER alpha and ER beta. However, there is only sparse human data regarding the relationship between dietary exposure of soy products containing phytoestrogens, such as genistein, and breast cancer risk. Therefore, the causative role of soy food intake in reducing breast cancer risk is still controversial.

- **Parabens.** Parabens are synthetic chemicals that are commonly used as preservatives in many foods—for example, beer, sauces, jams, and soft drinks. These chemicals appear as well in personal care products such as cosmetics. Parabens are absorbed through the skin and from the gastrointestinal tract and blood. Despite their relatively low toxicity profiles and a long history of safe uses, these chemicals are considered as potential carcinogens and endocrine disruptors because they can mimic estrogen in the body and disrupt the hormone balances.

Medical trials have revealed that the estrogenic properties of parabens (man-made chemicals) may perturb the mechanism of normal breast cells and potentially contribute to their abnormal growth and thus increase the risk of breast cancer. So far, there is only one study that reported the association of paraben exposures and breast cancer risk and mortality following breast cancer.

- **Per- and Polyfluoroalkyl/ Perfluorooctanoic acid/ Perfluorooctanoic acid. Per- and polyfluoroalkyl substances (PFAS)** are a group of man-made chemicals used in various industrial and consumer products. They are the

Microplastics (MPs)

Microplastics (MPs) are now a global issue due to increased plastic production, its use, and its constant discard. These tiny fragments, measuring less than 0.2 inches, represent significant threats to the environment and our health. These plastic fragments contain hazardous chemicals such as bisphenols, phthalates, and per- and poly-fluoroalkyl substances (PFAS). Recent research has uncovered a link between microplastics and cancer, prompting more investigation.

Studies demonstrate microplastics can infiltrate cells, disrupt biological processes, and potentially foster environments that promote cancer. In a study, the detrimental effects of *polypropylene microplastics* (PPMPs) on breast cancer metastasis were examined. The results suggest that PPMPs enhance metastasis-related gene expression and cytokines in breast cancer cells, exacerbating breast cancer spread. Furthermore, microplastics act as carriers for a range of contaminants, compounding their impact on human health.

most-studied PFAS, as are **perfluorooctanoic acid (PFOA)** and **perfluorooctane sulfonate (PFOS)**. They are considered as potential EDCs, since they have been shown to cause endocrine disruption by binding and activating the peroxisome proliferator activated receptor (PPAR)-α/γ signaling pathways, which then increases hepatic (liver) aromatase (an enzyme active in the conversion of testosterone to estrogen) concentrations and subsequent estrogen levels. Several studies found positive associations between breast cancer risk and these substances. However, a recent California Teachers case-control study showed no correlation of serum PFAS levels measured after diagnosis with breast cancer risk. More trials need to be conducted.

- **Polybrominated diphenyl ethers (PBDEs).** Polybrominated diphenyl ethers (PBDEs) are a group of synthetic halogenated compounds that have been widely distributed as environmental contaminants due to their extensive uses as additive flame retardants in household products, such as furniture, hard plastic coating in appliances, and more. There is a rising concern over the use of PBDEs in humans, as several animal studies have shown that PBDEs are able to cause endocrine disruptions and affect sexual and reproductive functions and developments. This is largely due to their interference with estrogen- and androgen-signaling pathways. High levels of PBDEs are consistently detected in human breast tissues. A recent study by Wei revealed a positive correlation of breast cancer growth with exposure to BDE-47, one of the PBDE's minor chemical constituents.

- **Polychlorinated biphenyls (PCBs).** Polychlorinated biphenyls (PCBs) are a halogenated aromatic group (chemicals which contain atoms of chloride, fluoride, bromide, and iodide) of ubiquitous, persistent environmental pollutants, and they can be present in high concentrations in fatty foods such as meat, fish, and dairy products. Like DTT and dioxins, these chemicals are *lipophilic* (combine with or dissolve in lipids or fats), bioaccumulate in adipose tissue, persistent in tissues, and are excreted in breast milk. In a review of epidemiological studies, the association between total PCBs and breast cancer risk were found to be *inconsistent*, regardless of the exposure measure. Again, more studies need to be done to further evaluate the PCBs and a possible relationship with breast cancer.

- **Polycyclic aromatic hydrocarbons (PAH).** Polycyclic aromatic hydrocarbons (PAH), synthetic fibers, organic solvents, oil mist, and insecticides. A potential relationship was also observed in the case of increased exposure to polycyclic aromatic hydrocarbons (PAH), synthetic fibers, organic solvents, oil mist, and insecticides.

- **Oral contraceptive pills.** Oral contraceptive pills that contain both *levonorgestrel* (a progestin) and *ethinyl estradiol* (an estrogen) are considered toxic EDCs. They alter normal reproductive function by mimicking the action of estrogen—and thus help to *prevent* normal hormone production. Due to wide availability and prevalent usage of oral contraceptives among women, there is considerable interest in investigating a possible link between contraceptive pill consumption and breast cancer risk.

Both prospective and retrospective studies identified an increased breast cancer risk associated with contraceptive pill usage, regardless of the type taken. A very recent study revealed that there was an increased risk of developing breast cancer—20 percent to 30 percent—in people who had used oral contraceptives. Part of this increase may be due to the progestin used (synthetic progesterone).

Kukasiewicz and his associates examined the medical literature concerning drugs that might constitute potential risk factors for breast cancer. These drugs were not synthetic hormone replacement drugs, and they found that antibiotics (prolonged intake of antibiotics, particularly *tetracyclines*), antidepressants (paroxetine, tricyclic antidepressants, and selective serotonin re-uptake inhibitors) might be associated with a greater risk of breast cancer. The data for statins, antihypertensive medications (for example, calcium channel blockers, angiotensin II-converting enzyme inhibitors) as well as NSAIDs (including aspirin ane ibuprofen) remains highly inconsistent. Therefore, more research needs to be done.

- **Phytoestrogens.** The chemicals that have been discussed so far are synthetic compounds that disrupt the endocrine system by mimicking or inhibiting endogenous hormones. However, there are also some naturally occurring chemicals that can mimic or inhibit the effects of endogenous hormones. *Phytoestrogens* are naturally occurring estrogens that can be found abundantly in plants. They are considered to be EDCs. In contrast to industrial or communal EDCs, some individuals believe that sometimes phytoestrogens can be beneficial, such as to treat and/or prevent breast cancer. Yet, negative effects associated with phytoestrogens were also reported. Lifelong exposure to estrogenic substances, especially during critical periods of development, can lead to severe long-term consequences from malignancies to abnormalities of the reproduction systems.

CONCLUSION

As you have seen, environmental toxins of all varieties, from toxic metals to endocrine disruptors, increase your risk of developing this major disease process. A Personalized Medicine specialist can measure toxic metals and many other toxins in the body, including endocrine disruptors. The great news is that the science is here to be able to remove lead, mercury, cadmium, and other toxic metals from your body. Excitedly, recent research has shown that removal of endocrine disruptors, including microplastics, from your system is no longer a thing of the past. (See Chapter 9, "Looking Forward," on page 264 for more information.)

And still, there are also a number of ways you can lower the exposure to these potentially cancer-promoting chemicals:

- Consuming more organic foods.

- Filtering your air with a science-backed filtration system.

- Purifying your water through filters.

- Switching to natural cleaning products.

- Using essential oils instead of synthetic fragrances.

- Using non-toxic skincare.

It can seem a bit overwhelming, but if you take it one step at a time, you can avoid many of these environmental risks. The power comes with knowing what to *avoid*.

6

Controllable Hormonal Risk Factors

Hormonal-related breast cancer is just as it sounds; breast cancer that is sensitive to hormones. It is estimated that approximately 70% of breast cancers are related to the receptors of two hormones—estrogen and progesterone. To understand your risk and benefits, it is important to understand how your hormones work in your body. There is a great deal of misinformation in the general community concerning hormones and their relationship to breast cancer. First, let's take a general look at your hormones and then we will more fully explore each hormone and their relationship to breast cancer.

WHAT IS A HORMONE?

We hear a lot about "hormones," but what are they, and why are they so important? *Hormones* are chemicals that are produced by our body's glands, organs, and tissues. There are over 50 different hormones that have been identified in the body, and each of these hormones helps control how our cells and organs work. Imagine a computer chip in a phone. Pull the chip out and the phone stops working. Put it back in, and you can start texting once again. Every one of our body's systems relies on our various hormones to function properly—from the beating of our hearts, to our ability to sleep or have babies. These hormonal molecules attach themselves to specific receptors on cells and tell the cells what they have to do. When the message they tell the cell is confusing or wrong, the behavior of the cell is likely to change—wherein a normal cell becomes an *abnormal* cell, dividing over and over and moving from one place to another. In addition, such behavior can weaken our immune system.

Another important factor to consider is the number of hormones produced in the body. The body will experience various health issues if there is an under-production, or over-production, of any one hormone. In addition, many of the hormones require a balance of other hormones to function properly. When they are imbalanced, they can create weight gain, mood swings, painful periods, low self-esteem, insomnia, skin problems, headache—and, yes, breast cancer.

Here is a quick look at eight hormones that play a part in developing breast cancer.

☐ *Estrogen*, along with progesterone, plays a major part in determining our sexual and reproductive roles. It is a key component as to whether you will develop breast cancer or not. But it is not just about estrogen. If you have estrogen, but not enough progesterone to keep it in balance, you have an increased risk of developing breast cancer. Because of estrogen's powerful effects, it is referred to as *estrogen dominance*. Moreover, this estrogen breakdown, known as *metabolization*, is also important. Your body breaks down estrogen into two major, and one minor, pathways. These pathways are a series of interconnected chemical interactions that regulate many functions within the body. If a pathway's process is abnormal, it can become another major risk factor for the development of breast cancer.

☐ *Progesterone* balances estrogen in the body; that is, it keeps the effects of estrogen in check. However, synthetic progesterone—called *progestin*—has been shown in several medical trials to increase one's risk of developing breast cancer. It is important to understand the difference between your body's own progesterone and the two other forms it comes in: *bioidentical* progesterone and *synthetic* progesterone. Unfortunately, the difference between bioidentical and synthetic progesterone is not commonly discussed with patients, nor is their respective increased risk of developing breast cancer if they take synthetic progesterone (progestin).

☐ *Testosterone* plays a key role in the development of male characteristics. However, it *also* plays a role in women's health and reproduction. There are some physicians who suggest giving testosterone to patients with low testosterone that have had breast cancer. It is vital to understand that it is all about balance when it comes to the hormones in your body. If you no longer have estrogen (due to your treatment for breast cancer), then you should not have testosterone replaced, even if the levels are low, since you will *then* have a significantly increased risk of developing heart disease. In addition, many women have high testosterone levels. This disease process is called *polycystic ovarian syndrome* (PCOS). Women with PCOS tend to commonly have high insulin levels, which is a risk factor for breast cancer as well as type 2 diabetes, obesity, and cardiovascular disease.

☐ *Dehydroepiandrosterone* (*DHEA*) makes estrogen and testosterone in the body, and it also balances cortisol (which is your stress hormone). If you have had hormonal-related breast cancer, it is not recommended to replace DHEA in the body since it makes estrogen. However, if you are trying to prevent breast cancer and your DHEA levels are low or suboptimal, replacement of DHEA is recommended to build your immune system to prevent getting breast cancer. It is also a powerful anti-inflammatory agent.

☐ *Cortisol* is your *stress* hormone, and it is balanced by DHEA in your body. You must have cortisol to live, or you will pass away in only seven days. In addition, one of the main functions of cortisol in the body is to build your immune system and to decrease inflammation.

☐ *Insulin* is your hormone that regulates your blood sugar. If insulin is not working effectively in your body, you have an elevated risk of developing breast cancer as well as an increased risk of weight gain, which is in itself a controllable risk factor for the development of cancer of the breast.

☐ *Melatonin* is commonly looked at as your *sleep* hormone, but it also has great immune-building properties. Likewise, melatonin is also a key therapy for breast cancer and to help prevent a reoccurrence.

☐ *Thyroid hormones* play many important roles in your body that affect nearly every organ and cell in your body. If your body produces too little thyroid hormone (*hypothyroidism*) or too much thyroid hormone (*hyperthyroidism*), you have an increased risk of developing breast cancer.

Each of these hormones will be looked at along with their relationship to the prevention of breast cancer, as well as their association if they are not balanced, to developing breast cancer.

NATURAL ESTROGEN

Estrogen is a hormone that is produced mainly in the ovaries. Smaller amounts are produced in the adrenal glands, fats cells, liver, heart, skin, brain, and placenta during pregnancy. It is essential to a woman's sexual development. There are receptor sites for estrogen practically everywhere in the human body: in the brain, muscles, bone, bladder, gut, uterus, ovaries, vagina, breasts, eyes, heart, lungs, and blood vessels, to name a few. Estrogen plays over 400 crucial roles in the body.

FUNCTIONS OF ESTROGEN IN YOUR BODY

- Acts as a natural calcium blocker to keep your arteries open

- Aids in the formation of neurotransmitters in your brain—such as serotonin—which decrease depression, irritability, anxiety, and pain sensitivity

- Decreases LDL (*bad* cholesterol) and prevents its oxidation

- Decreases lipoprotein A (a risk factor of heart disease)

- Decreases the accumulation of plaque on your arteries

- Decreases wrinkles

- Decreases your risk of developing colon cancer

- Dilates your small arteries

- Enhances energy

- Enhances magnesium uptake and utilization

- Enhances the production of nerve-growth factor

- Helps maintain the elasticity of your arteries

- Helps maintain your memory

- Helps to prevent Alzheimer's disease

- Helps prevent muscle damage and maintains muscles

- Helps prevent tooth loss

- Helps regulate blood pressure

- Helps with fine motor skills

- Improves insulin sensitivity

- Improves mood

- Increases blood flow

- Increases concentration

- Increases HDL (*good* cholesterol) by 10 to 15 percent

- Increases reasoning ability

- Increases sexual interest

- Increases the water content of your skin, which is responsible for your skin's thickness and softness

- Increases your metabolic rate, which helps your body run at a youthful level

- Inhibits platelet stickiness, which decreases your risk of heart disease

- Lowers homocysteine (a risk factor for heart disease)

- Maintains bone density

- Maintains the amount of collagen in your skin

- Protects against endothelial dysfunction by increasing endothelial nitric oxide

- Protects against macular degeneration, an age-related eye ailment that may cause vision loss

- Reduces vascular proliferation and inflammatory responses, which decreases your risk of heart disease

- Reduces your overall risk of heart disease by 40 to 50 percent

- Reduces your risk of cataracts

- Regulates body temperature

SIGNS AND SYMPTOMS OF ESTROGEN DEFICIENCY

☐ Acne

☐ Anxiety

☐ Arthritis

☐ Bladder problems (more infections, urinary leakage)

☐ Brittle hair and nails

☐ Chronic fatigue

☐ Decrease in breast size

☐ Decrease in dexterity

☐ Decrease in memory and focus

☐ Decrease in sexual interest/function

☐ Depression

☐ Diabetes/insulin resistance

☐ Difficulty losing weight, even with diet and exercise

☐ Dry eye

☐ Elevated cholesterol

☐ Fibromyalgia

☐ Food cravings

☐ Heart attack

☐ Hypertension/ elevated blood pressure

☐ Increase in facial hair

☐ Increase in insulin resistance, which can lead to diabetes

☐ Increase in tension headaches

☐ Increased cholesterol

☐ Infertility

☐ Joint pain

☐ Low energy, especially at the end of the day

☐ More frequent migraines

☐ More wrinkles (aging skin)

☐ Oily skin

☐ Osteoporosis/ osteopenia

☐ Panic attacks

☐ Polycystic ovarian syndrome

☐ Restless sleep

☐ Stress incontinence

☐ Strokes

☐ Thinner skin

☐ Thinning hair

☐ Urinary stress incontinence/ leakage

☐ Urinary tract infections

☐ Vaginal dryness

☐ Vulvodynia (vaginal pain)

☐ Weight gain around the middle

Most young women who suffer estrogen-related problems are estrogen-dominant. However, as women grow older, most develop estrogen deficiency. It is extremely important that estrogen be replaced when it declines after menopause, provided you do not have a hormonal-related breast cancer, since many studies have shown that estrogen helps to prevent heart disease and cognitive decline. In addition, not all women lose estrogen at menopause. Estrogen is stored in fat cells; therefore, if a woman is overweight, she may not need estrogen for several years after she stops cycling.

CAUSES OF ESTROGEN DEFICIENCY

- Hormonal dysregulation following delivery
- Hypothalamic dysfunction
- Hypothyroidism
- Insulin resistance
- Perimenopause/menopause
- Pituitary dysfunction
- Polycystic ovarian syndrome (PCOS)
- Premature ovarian decline/ premature ovarian failure
- Synthetic hormone replacement
- Turner syndrome

Estrogen levels are lower in women who smoke. This may be why women who smoke experience more menopausal symptoms than women who do not smoke. In addition, low-fat diets decrease free estrogen (the amount of estrogen available for the body to use).

SIGNS AND SYMPTOMS OF EXCESS ESTROGEN

- ☐ Bloating
- ☐ Brain fog
- ☐ Cervical dysplasia
- ☐ Decrease in sexual interest
- ☐ Depression with anxiety or agitation
- ☐ Elevated risk of developing breast cancer
- ☐ Fatigue
- ☐ Fibrocystic breasts
- ☐ Headaches
- ☐ Heavy periods
- ☐ Hypothyroidism (increases the binding of thyroid hormone, which causes low thyroid hormone levels)
- ☐ Increased risk of developing autoimmune diseases
- ☐ Increased risk of developing uterine cancer
- ☐ Irritability
- ☐ Mood swings
- ☐ Panic attacks
- ☐ Poor sleep
- ☐ Swollen breasts

☐ Uterine fibroids (non-cancerous tumors of the uterus)

☐ Water retention

☐ Weight gain (especially in the abdomen, hips, and thighs)

CAUSES OF EXCESS ESTROGEN

- Diet low in grains and fiber
- Environmental estrogens
- Excessive doses of estrogen replacement therapy
- Foods that can increase your estrogen level
- Impaired elimination of estrogen through the liver/GI tract
- Lack of exercise

Methods That Can Lower Excess Estrogen Levels

- Exercise
- Improve phase I and phase II detoxification of the liver
- Lose weight if you are overweight
- Lower your dose of estrogen replacement
- Phase III detoxification of your gut (GI tract)

THREE TYPES OF NATURAL ESTROGENS

Your body makes many forms of estrogen. The first is estrogen (E1), which is produced after menopause. The second is estradiol (E2), formed during our reproductive years, and the third is estradiol (E3, formed during pregnancy).

ESTRONE (E1)

Although serum estradiol (E2) levels decrease significantly after natural menopause, a considerable amount of estrone (E1) still exists in women after this phase of life. It is derived from estradiol. High levels of E1 stimulate breast and uterine tissue, and many researchers believe this action increases the risks of developing breast cancer and uterine cancer.

E1 is considered a reserve source for estrogen. If your estrogen levels get too low, your body can draw from and use this stored amount. Estrone produced in adipose tissues may have a role in modulating the loss of bone mass occurring after menopause.

Before menopause, E1 is made by your ovaries, adrenal glands, liver, and fat cells. It is converted into E2 in your ovaries. After menopause, very little E1 becomes E2 since the ovaries stop working. In later years, E1 is made in your fat cells and, to a lesser degree, in your liver and adrenal glands. Therefore, the more body fat you have, the more E1 you make. Consequently, obese women tend to have an increased E1-to-E2 ratio. In addition, routine alcohol consumption decreases ovarian hormone levels and increases levels of E1, which can lead to an increased risk of breast cancer.

ESTRADIOL (E2)

Estradiol is the strongest form of estrogen. It is twelve times stronger than E1, and eighty times stronger than estriol (E3). It is the main estrogen produced by the body before menopause. Most of your body's E2 is made in your ovaries. High levels of E2 are associated with an increased risk of breast and uterine cancer.

FUNCTIONS OF E2 IN YOUR BODY

- Decreases fatigue
- Decreases LDL (*bad* cholesterol)
- Decreases platelet stickiness
- Decreases total cholesterol
- Decreases triglycerides (transdermal, on the skin, administration of E2 only)
- Helps maintain memory
- Helps maintain potassium levels

- Helps maintain your bones
- Helps with the absorption of calcium, magnesium, and zinc
- Improves sleep
- Increases endorphins
- Increases growth hormone
- Increases HDL (*good* cholesterol)
- Increases serotonin
- Works as an antioxidant

E2 is the form of estrogen you lose at menopause. However, two-thirds of postmenopausal women up to the age of eighty continue to make some E2. Women who have had a surgical procedure that affected their ovaries tend to have lower levels of E2 than other women.

SIGNS AND SYMPTOMS OF ESTRADIOL DECLINE

☐ Aching joints

☐ Anxiety attacks that worsen around menstrual cycle

☐ Bladder changes, such as more infections, pain during urination, more frequent urination, and urinary leakage

☐ Bone loss in spine, resulting in slumped posture

☐ Decline in collagen, resulting in dry, crawly, looser skin and more wrinkles

☐ Difficulty having an orgasm

☐ Difficulty losing weight, even with diet and exercise

☐ Dry, brittle nails

☐ Dry eye

☐ Fibromyalgia pain syndrome

☐ Food cravings

☐ Increase in facial hair

☐ Increase in tension headaches

☐ Loss of energy, or feeling too tired to get through the day

☐ Loss of sexual interest

☐ Memory and concentration problems that worsen before menstruation

☐ Mood swings, episodic tearfulness for no reason, irritability, angry outbursts, and spells of depression (especially pre-menstrual)

☐ More irritable bowel problems prior to and during menstruation

☐ Muscle soreness or stiffness

☐ Palpitations, especially those that get worse a few days prior to menstruation and during the cycle

☐ Premenstrual migraines or more frequent migraines

☐ Restless sleep, difficulty sleeping (especially prior to menstruating), or multiple awakenings during the night

☐ Spiking blood pressure (or blood pressure that is higher than normal)

☐ Thinner hair and more scalp hair loss

☐ Vaginal dryness, resulting in pain during intercourse

☐ Weight gain around the middle

☐ Worsening allergies, such as sensitivities to chemicals or perfumes

☐ Worsening PMS

ESTRIOL (E3)

Estriol (E3) has a much less stimulatory effect on the breast and uterine lining than E1 or E2. E3 does not promote breast cancer. In fact, considerable evidence exists to show that it protects against breast cancer. In Western Europe, E3 has been used for this purpose for over 60 years.

Estrogen has two main receptor sites to which it binds in the body: estrogen receptor-alpha and estrogen receptor-beta. Estrogen receptor-alpha increases cell growth and estrogen receptor-beta decreases cell growth, helps to prevent breast cancer development, and promotes beneficial estrogenic effects on skin, bone, brain, and other tissues. E2 equally activates estrogen receptors alpha and beta. E1 activates estrogen receptor-alpha selectively at a ratio of five-to-one. Therefore, E1 prefers to bind with the alpha receptor type, which increases cell proliferation. In contrast, E3 binds preferentially to estrogen receptor-beta at a three-to-one ratio. It is believed that this selective binding to estrogen-beta receptor sites imparts to E3 a potential for breast cancer prevention.

Studies over the last forty years have revealed that E3, given experimentally to women with breast cancer, has decreased a reoccurrence of the disease. This includes one study in the 1970s in which women with metastatic breasts were given E3. Of the women, 37 percent experienced remission—their cancer did not spread any further.

However, E3 does not offer the bone, heart, or brain protection that E2 provides. E3 does, however, have some positive effects on heart health by lowering cholesterol. It is also effective in controlling symptoms of menopause, including hot flashes, vaginal dryness, and frequent urinary tract infections (UTIs). It also is used to help treat osteoporosis, cancer, vascular disease, and multiple sclerosis. In fact, increased levels of estriol have been linked to improvements in cognition.

I usually begin by prescribing 20 percent E2 and 80 percent E3 for an estrogen prescription if tests reveal that a patient's estrogen levels are low. Then the percentages of E2 and E3 are adjusted according to lab results of each patient. The combination of E2 and E3 together is called "biest," which is a prescription that a compounding pharmacist (a pharmacist who puts together medications in customized dosages) can formulate for you. Any percentage of these two estrogens can be used, since the dosage is personalized.

Hormone Testing

There are four ways to measure hormones and their breakdown products:

- **Salivary (or saliva testing)** is the preferred method of hormone testing. It is a non-invasive method of testing and can be done in the privacy of your own home. Saliva testing is the measurement of the bioavailable hormone; in other words, the amount of the hormone that is available for the body to use. Saliva testing is also the best way to measure hormones that are applied on the skin, such as estrogen and testosterone. In addition, cortisol (your stress hormone) must be measured by saliva, since it is the "gold standard" in medicine. Published research has confirmed the accuracy of saliva testing in determining the values of all three estrogens, progesterone, testosterone, DHEA, cortisol, and melatonin. When compared with serum, saliva testing is also more cost-effective.

- **Blood testing (serum testing)** measures the bound hormone, plus the free hormone, in the body. Therefore, it measures both the inactive and active forms. In addition, as previously mentioned, serum testing has been shown not to be as accurate for hormones that are applied to the skin since they are underestimated in the blood. Consequently, if your healthcare provider uses blood testing to measure your hormones, you can easily be overdosed.

- **Urine testing** measures the downstream metabolites, or the breakdown products of the hormones. It is not a direct measurement of the hormones in your body and therefore cannot be used for dosing hormones. Urine testing, however, is very important to evaluate how your body is breaking down each hormone particularly estrogen. An increase in the 4-hydroxyestrone (4-OH estrone) form of estrogen increases your risk of developing breast cancer.

- **Blood spot testing** is a form of collection in which you place blood drops on a filter card after a finger prick with a lancet. Once the blood has dried, blood spot cards are extremely stable for shipment. Research has shown that blood spot testing is more accurate than serum for measuring blood hormone levels in patients with topically applied hormones.

FUNCTIONS OF E3 IN YOUR BODY

- Benefits the vaginal lining

- Blocks E1 by occupying the estrogen receptor sites on your breast cells

- Controls symptoms of menopause, including hot flashes, insomnia, and vaginal dryness

- Decreases LDL (*bad* cholesterol)

- Helps reduce pathogenic bacteria

- Helps restore the proper pH of the vagina, which prevents urinary tract infections (UTIs)

- Helps your gut maintain a favorable environment for the growth of good bacteria (lactobacilli)

- Increases HDL (*good* cholesterol)

Before you begin hormone replacement therapy [HRT], it is necessary that you have your levels of all three estrogens measured. You should also have them measured regularly thereafter; to help your healthcare provider ensure you maintain the optimal amount of each type of estrogen. (See the *Hormone Testing* inset on page 111.)

ESTROGEN DETOXIFICATION

Estrogen synthesis, estrogen metabolism, and estrogen detoxification are of paramount importance in order to maintain optimal health, prevent breast cancer, and to also prevent your developing this disease again. The effect of estrogen on your body is not related solely to its function but also to how it is detoxified in the liver and in other tissues.

Toxins are poisonous substances that are either produced by the body, inhaled, or ingested. When they build up, the health effects can be quite serious. This is why it is important to detoxify.

Detoxification is the process through which toxic substances—environmental pollutants, medications, byproducts of metabolism, and more—are removed from the body. This process is one of the major functions of the liver, gastrointestinal tract, kidneys, and skin, with the liver being one of the most important organs of detoxification. Studies have shown that the effectiveness of the body's ability to break down toxins varies from person to person.

Each year, over 2.5 billion pounds of pesticides are dumped on croplands, forests, lawns, and fields. According to the US Environmental Protection Agency, more than 4 billion pounds of chemicals were released into the ground in the year 2000, threatening our natural groundwater sources.

Toxin Buildup

Toxicity can affect your endocrine, neurological, and immune systems. Endocrine toxicity affects reproduction, menstruation, libido, metabolic rate, stress tolerance, and glucose regulation. Immune toxicity may be a factor in asthma, allergies, skin disorders, chronic infections, and cancer. Neurological toxicity also affects cognition, mood, and neurological function.

SIGNS AND SYMPTOMS OF TOXIN BUILDUP

☐ Allergies

☐ Bloating

☐ Chemical sensitivities

☐ Clammy hands

☐ Constipation

☐ Depression

☐ Difficulty tolerating exercise

☐ Disturbed sleep

☐ Fatigue

☐ Flatulence

☐ Fluid retention

☐ Headaches

☐ Intolerance to fat, alcohol, and caffeine

☐ Irritability

☐ Itchy skin

☐ Jaundice (eyes and skin may be yellow in severe cases)

☐ Lethargy

☐ Muscle aches and pains

☐ Nausea

☐ Trouble breathing

Some Situations That Can Increase Your Exposure to Toxins

There are some situations that can increase your exposure to toxins:

- Chronic infections
- Chronic inflammation
- Chronic use of medication
- Drinking tap water
- Excessive consumption of alcohol
- Excessive consumption of caffeine
- Excessive consumption of processed food and fats
- Intestinal (gut) dysfunction
- Kidney problems
- Lack of exercise
- Liver dysfunction
- Living or working near areas of high traffic of industrial plants
- Occupational or other exposure to pesticides, paints, or other toxic substances without adequate protective equipment

- Recreational drug use
- Tobacco use

- Using pesticides, paint, or other toxic substances without adequate protective gear

In addition to the previous issues, genetic factors and aging can also affect your liver's ability to detoxify the body.

In terms of exposure to toxins, you are exposed to estrogen-like compounds every day. These chemicals, known as *xenoestrogens*, are found in drugs, plastics, and cleaning products. Xenoestrogens have estrogenic activity and can interfere with, or mimic, your own hormone synthesis. Consequently, they can be disruptive to your own hormone production. (See Chapter 5, "Controllable Environmental Risk Factors," page 92.)

THE DETOXIFICATION PROCESS

Detoxification is a process by which your body transforms toxins and medications into harmless molecules that can be eliminated. This process takes place primarily in the liver and to a smaller degree in other tissues, such as your gastrointestinal tract, skin, kidneys, and lungs.

There are three major phases of detoxification that your body undergoes. The first two take place in your liver. In phase I, enzymes change toxins into intermediate compounds. In phase II, the intermediate compounds are neutralized through the addition of a water-soluble molecule. Phase III is accomplished by multiple organ systems—namely, your gut, kidneys, and lymphatic system, after which the body is able to eliminate the transformed toxins through urine or feces.

It is very important for you to detoxify estrogen completely in your body. The good news is that all three phases of detoxification can be measured to see if your liver and GI tract are able to adequately detoxify substances.

■ Phase I Detoxification: Your First Line of Defense

In phase I detoxification, enzymes in the cytochrome P450 (CYP) system use oxygen to modify toxic compounds, medications, and steroid hormones. This is your first line of defense for the detoxification of all environmental toxins, medications, supplements (for example, vitamins), and many waste products that your body produces.

The cytochrome P450 (CYP) system is a group of over sixty enzymes that your body uses to break down toxins. Most of these enzymes are located in your liver. Three of the twelve cytochrome P450 gene families share the main responsibility for drug metabolism in your body. In other words, many of the medications that you take are broken down through this system. The cytochrome P450 system is also involved in other processes in your body, such as the conversion of vitamin D into more active forms.

Phase I occurs in the liver, where estrogen goes through the cytochrome P450 system. This influences the amount of estrogen that is exposed to your other cells. If you do not completely detoxify the intermediates of estrogen metabolism, it can result in an increase in estrogen activity in your body.

Within your own genetic makeup, there are variations called *single nucleotide polymorphisms* (SNPs, pronounced "snips"). These SNPs in your genes code for a particular enzyme that can increase or decrease the activity of that enzyme. Both increased and decreased activity may be harmful to you. Furthermore, if you increase phase I clearance (elimination) without increasing phase II clearance, it can lead to a buildup of intermediates that may be more toxic than the original substance.

Decreased phase I clearance will cause toxic accumulation in your body. Sometimes, the body completes phase I but builds up a toxic metabolite that phase II is unable to eliminate from the system. Adverse reactions to medications are often due to a decreased capacity for clearing them from your system.

Nutrients Required for Phase I Detoxification

- Copper
- Flavonoids
- Folic acid
- Magnesium
- Niacin
- Vitamin B_2
- Vitamin B_3
- Vitamin B_6
- Vitamin B_{12}
- Vitamin C
- Zinc

▥ Phase II Detoxification: Conjugation of Toxins

In phase II detoxification, large water-soluble molecules are added to toxins, usually at the reactive site formed by phase I reactions. After phase II modifications, the body is able to eliminate the transformed toxins in the urine or the feces. Phase II detoxification has six stages.

Stage I: *Glutathione conjugation.* Glutathione is the strongest antioxidant that your body makes. It plays an important role in the detoxification of carcinogens and other environmental toxins. This stage of detoxification requires glutathione and vitamin B_6.

Stage II: *Amino acid conjugation.* In this stage, amino acids combine with toxins to neutralize them. Glycine and taurine are amino acids used for this pathway, along with glutamine, arginine, and ornithine.

Stage III: *Methylation.* Methylation is needed for many reactions in the body, including detoxification of estrogen and breakdown of homocysteine. It requires folic acid, choline, methionine, trimethylglycine (TMG), and S-Adenosyl methionine (SAMe).

Stage IV: *Sulfation.* The sulfation pathway is required in the detoxification of food additives, steroid hormones, thyroid hormones, estrogen hormones, and toxins from intestinal bacteria. It requires cysteine, methionine, and molybdenum.

Stage V: *Acetylation.* The acetylation pathway detoxifies substances known as amines, such as histamine and tyramine, as well as compounds such as caffeine and choline. It requires acetyl coenzyme A (acetyl-CoA) and vitamin B_5. Sluggish acetylation has been associated with an increased risk of bladder cancer.

Stage VI: *Glucuronidation.* This pathway is responsible for metabolizing drugs and estrogens and also conjugates bilirubin. It requires glucuronic acid. Calcium D-glucarate supports the glucuronidation pathways and metabolism of estrogen.

◼ Phase III Detoxification: Antiporter System

Recent scientific study suggests the existence of a third detoxification phase, which is located primarily in the small intestine. It is called the antiporter system, or simply phase III, and makes use of antiporter proteins for its detoxification activity. These proteins can be increased (boosting detoxification) or inhibited, *decreasing* detoxification. The most studied of these proteins is known as P-glycoprotein 1 (P-gp).

P-glycoprotein is found in the intestines, liver, kidneys, and capillary endothelial cells, which form the blood-brain barrier (BBB) and blood-testis barrier (BTB). It helps in the elimination of toxins from these areas of the body.

Inflammation of the gut can hinder the functioning of phase III, leading to a decrease in the functioning of phase II and then a buildup of the metabolites created in phase I. This domino effect can result in oxidative damage and impair your body's entire detoxification system. In light of this fact, in order to evaluate your body's ability to rid itself of dangerously high levels of certain substances—including estrogen—a phase I/phase II liver detoxification test and a gastrointestinal (GI) health test should be performed. Fostering a healthy GI tract and reducing inflammation in the gut allows your detoxification system to bind toxins and eliminate them.

SYNTHETIC ESTROGEN

Estrogen replacement comes in many forms. The most commonly prescribed hormone replacement in the world remains a drug that contains horse estrogens (*equilin* and *equilenin*) and additives that are synthetic. These additives and coatings may cause their own side effects, including a burning sensation in the urinary tract, allergies, joint aches, and an increased risk of developing breast cancer. This form of estrogen is taken by mouth.

How you take estrogen is also important. I recommend using estrogen by the transdermal route, which means applying it to the skin. Estrogen used vaginally is also an effective form. Orally used estrogen, by comparison, can have major side effects.

SIDE EFFECTS OF TAKING ESTROGEN ORALLY

- Decrease in growth hormone (the hormone that keeps you younger)
- Elevated liver enzymes
- Increase in C-reactive protein (CRP), a marker of inflammation
- Increase in gallstones

DECREASE INFLAMMATION

- Increase in sex hormone-binding globulin (SHBG), which can decrease testosterone
- Increased blood pressure
- Increased carbohydrate cravings
- Increased estrone (E1)
- Increased prothrombotic effects (blood clots)
- Increased triglycerides
- Interruption in metabolism of tryptophan and serotonin (neurotransmitters that keep you calm and happy)
- Weight gain

Estrogen creams are the preferred method of replacing this hormone, which has so many functions. Many studies have been conducted on transdermal application of estradiol (E2). One study revealed that, when compared with no hormone therapy, the use of oral-conjugated equine estrogen or oral estradiol was associated with excess risk of venous thromboembolism (blood clot). In contrast, the use of transdermal estradiol was not associated with excess venous thromboembolism.

When applied, it is important that you rub the estrogen in for two minutes and rotate sites. Discuss with your healthcare practitioner the best location on your skin to apply the estrogen, since it is best absorbed when applied to areas that contain fat cells—*except* for the abdomen.

Detoxification and Nutrition

The detoxification process is dependent on nutrients. All three phases of detoxification are fueled by vitamins, minerals, and other key food components. Therefore, if you are undernourished and lack key vitamins or nutrients, you may not be able to break down estrogen properly. In addition, if your GI tract is not functioning optimally, you will not metabolize estrogen effectively. This can leave estrogen available to cause cell transformation in the breasts and predispose you to breast cancer. Consequently, adequate nutrition is essential for effective detoxification.

ESTROGEN METABOLISM (BREAKDOWN)

If estrogen is metabolized (broken down) poorly in your body, it is one of the main risk factors for the development of breast cancer.

Estrogen Metabolism

Estrogen is broken down into two major pathways, the 2-OH and 16-OH estrogen along with the minor pathway the 4-OH estrogen. The 2-OH is the "good estrogen." Methoxy estrogens, including *2-methoxyestradiol* (types of estrogen), have been shown to inhibit cancer development by suppressing cell growth and estrogen oxidation due to effects on microtubules, which help support and shape cell stabilization. It also has anti-metastatic activity by inhibiting cell replication.

Your body needs a small amount of 16-OH estrogen to maintain bone structure, but it has significant strong estrogenic activity. Studies have shown that high levels of 16-OH relate to an increased risk in the development of breast cancer. Elevated levels of 16-OH estrogen are associated with obesity, hypothyroidism, pesticide toxicity, omega-6 fatty acid excess, and inflammatory cytokines. Results of a prospective study support the hypothesis that the estrogen metabolism pathway favoring 2-hydroxylation over 16 alpha-hydroxylation is associated with a reduced risk of invasive breast cancer risk in premenopausal women.

If your body breaks down estrogen into mostly the 4-OH form, it directly damages DNA and causes mutations. Therefore, the 4-OH form is proposed to enhance breast cancer development. Synthetic estrogens commonly increase metabolism into the 4-OH estrone.

Fortunately, by improving methylation (see page 119) and using other nutrients, you can have a normal 4-OH level.

THERAPEUTIC BENEFITS OF ESTROGEN

The benefits of estrogen are many. It can help to prevent or improve many disease processes. Estrogen helps maintain memory, prevent heart disease, helps the body repair, and helps your body maintain the youthfulness of the skin. It also lowers your blood sugar. Above all else, estrogen is anti-inflammatory.

In addition to these benefits, estrogen can also strengthen your immune system. Research suggests that estrogen deficiency puts you in a state of accelerated aging. Furthermore, a meta-analysis of twenty-seven studies showed a 28 percent reduction in mortality in menopausal women under age sixty who used hormone replacement therapy (HRT). The participants also displayed improved quality of life.

Unfortunately, the study known as the "Study of Women's Health Across the Nation" revealed the number of women with low estrogen to be greater than previously thought. In light of their findings, the authors of this study proposed the use of estrogen replacement therapy (ERT).

PROGESTERONE

Progesterone is one of your sex hormones. It plays a role in menstruation, pregnancy, and the formation of embryos. Progesterone is made in the ovaries up until menopause. After menopause, it is made in the adrenal glands. Progesterone is made from pregnenolone and performs many functions in your body. In addition, progesterone works together with estrogen in your body to help you achieve optimal hormonal balance.

FUNCTIONS OF PROGESTERONE IN YOUR BODY

- Acts as a diuretic
- Acts as an anti-inflammatory
- Aids in ovulation
- Balances estrogen

- Effects the potentiation of GABA
- Enhances the action of thyroid hormones
- Has a positive effect on sleep
- Helps build bone
- Helps maintain bladder function
- Helps prevent anxiety, irritability, and mood swings
- Helps promote implantation of the egg
- Helps restore proper cell-oxygen levels
- Helps the body use and eliminate fats
- Helps to maintain pregnancy
- Increases metabolic rate

- Increases scalp hair
- Induces conversion of E1 to inactive E1S form
- Lowers LDL (*bad* cholesterol)
- Modulates oxytocin receptor binding in the hypothalamus
- Promotes T helper type 2 (Th2) immunity
- Promotes the formation of myelin sheaths
- Protects breast health
- Relaxes smooth muscle
- Relaxes the smooth muscle of the gut to aid in breaking down food
- Supports immune system

Progesterone levels in the body can drop below optimal levels at different times in your life. There are many reasons why this can happen. (See the "Causes of Progesterone Deficiency" list on page 121). When progesterone levels decline, there can be side effects, some more serious than others. A study measured blood levels of progesterone in almost 6,000 women that were premenopausal. Women with the highest levels of progesterone who had regular cycles had an 88 percent reduction in the risk of developing breast cancer. In another study, over 1,000 women who had undergone treatment for infertility were evaluated for over thirty years. The trial was done to look at subsequent breast cancer risk. Women who were deficient in progesterone had a 5.4-times increased risk of developing premenopausal breast cancer and were ten times as likely to die from any cancer.

SIGNS AND SYMPTOMS OF PROGESTERONE DEFICIENCY

☐ Anxiety

☐ Decreased high-density lipoprotein (HDL) levels

☐ Decreased libido

☐ Depression

☐ Excessive menstruation (lasting longer than seven days, with very heavy bleeding)

☐ Hypersensitivity

☐ Insomnia

☐ Irritability

☐ Migraine headaches prior to menstrual cycles

☐ Mood swings

☐ Nervousness

☐ Osteoporosis

☐ Pain and inflammation

☐ Weight gain

CAUSES OF PROGESTERONE DEFICIENCY

As mentioned, progesterone deficiency may be caused by a variety of factors.

- Aging
- Antidepressants
- Deficiencies of vitamins A, B_6, C, and zinc
- Excessive arginine consumption
- High sugar intake
- Hypothyroidism (decreased thyroid hormone)
- Impaired production
- Increased production of prolactin
- Low luteinizing hormone (LH)
- Saturated fat intake
- Stress

SIGNS AND SYMPTOMS OF EXCESS PROGESTERONE

Just as your body can have too much estrogen, it can also have too much progesterone. Too much progesterone can lead to a variety of side effects.

☐ Anxiety

☐ Decreased glucose tolerance, which can lead to an increase in blood sugar

☐ Decreased growth hormone

☐ Incontinence (leaky bladder)

☐ Increased appetite

☐ Increased carbohydrate cravings

☐ Increased cortisol

☐ Increased fat storage and weight gain

☐ Increased insulin and insulin resistance

☐ Increased the risk of gallstones

☐ Irritability

☐ Laxity of ligaments to relax, which can lead to backaches, leg aches, and achy hips

☐ Mood swings

☐ Relaxation of smooth muscles of the gut, which may cause bloating, fullness, or constipation

☐ Suppressed immune system

Unlike excess estrogen, which can be caused by a variety of factors, high progesterone levels occur less commonly—the major reason this happens is due to too high a dose of progesterone being prescribed by a healthcare provider.

BIOIDENTICAL PROGESTERONE

Bioidentical progesterone, also called natural progesterone, means that the progesterone has the same chemical structure as the progesterone that you were born with, but it is created using natural ingredients. Synthetic progesterone, which is chemically different, will be discussed on page 123, but it is *not* the same chemical structure.

Bioidentical progesterone, since it is biologically identical to the progesterone produced by the human body, has plenty of good effects not seen with synthetic progesterone. Consequently, many of these properties are similar to the ones that are produced by the body itself.

EFFECTS OF BIOIDENTICAL PROGESTERONE

- Balances estrogen levels
- Balances fluids in the cells
- Decreases the rate of cancer on all progesterone receptors
- Does not change the good effect estrogen has on blood flow
- Enhances the action of thyroid hormones
- Has a natural calming effect
- Helps restore effective cell oxygen levels
- Helps you sleep
- Helps your body use and eliminate fats
- Increases beneficial effects estrogen has on blood vessel dilation (hardened arteries)
- Increases metabolic rate
- Increases scalp hair
- Induces conversion of E1 to the inactive E1S form (E1S does not increase the risk of breast cancer)
- Is a natural antidepressant
- Is a natural diuretic (water pill)
- Is an anti-inflammatory
- Leaves the body quickly
- Lowers cholesterol
- Lowers high blood pressure
- May protect against breast cancer by inhibiting breast tissue overgrowth
- Normalizes and improves libido
- Prevents migraine headaches that are menstrual cycle-related

- Promotes a healthy immune system
- Promotes myelination, which helps protect nerves from injury

- Relaxes smooth muscle
- Stimulates the production of new bone

One of the most commonly asked questions about hormones is: Does bioidentical increase the risk of developing breast cancer? Studies have shown that progesterone does not induce estrogen-stimulated breast cell proliferation (growth). In fact, bioidentical progesterone has been shown in clinical trials to decrease the risk of developing breast cancer. One study looked at 80,000 postmenopausal women who used different kinds of hormone replacement therapy over eight years. It found that women who had used estrogen in combination with synthetic progestin had a 69 percent increased risk of developing breast cancer when compared with women who had never taken HRT.

Women who had used progesterone in combination with estrogen had no increased risk of developing breast cancer when compared with women who had not used HRT, and they *also* had a decreased risk of developing breast cancer when compared with women who had used progestin. Another study done by the same researchers found a 40 percent increased risk of developing breast cancer in women who had used estrogen with progestin. In women who had used estrogen combined with progesterone, there was a trend toward a decreased risk of developing breast cancer.

SYNTHETIC PROGESTERONE

Synthetic progesterone is called *progestin*. It is very different from bioidentical progesterone since it does not have the same chemical structure as the progesterone that your body makes on its own. Consequently, progestins do not reproduce the actions of bioidentical progesterone (which have similar effects on the body as the progesterone the body produces itself). For example, progestins do not help balance the estrogen in the body. They interfere with the body's production of progesterone and may attach themselves to many of your body's receptor sites, not just the progesterone receptors. Furthermore, progestins stop the protective effects estrogen has on your heart and can cause spasms of your arteries.

There are now many studies that show that progestins increase breast cancer replication and growth due to the stimulation of estrogen receptors by progestin, supporting the research that progestins increase the risk of breast cancer. In addition, one study revealed that estrogen plus progestin increases

What Is HRT?

Hormone replacement therapy (HRT) is a form of hormone therapy used to treat symptoms associated with hormonal imbalances in women. It is also used to help prevent disease. Up until a few decades ago, the only hormone replacement therapy available in the United States and most countries was synthetic hormone replacement.

Synthetic HRT

Some people may hear the word *synthetic* and think of another word—*fake*—but this is not always the case. When it comes to hormone replacement, the word *synthetic* means that the chemical structure is not what your own body makes. Conversely, *natural* (when referring to hormones) means the *exact same* chemical structure that your body produces. It does not mean that the item has a plant origin, even though hormones are made from soy or yams. If the chemical structure of the hormone matches the chemical structure of the hormone in your body, it is called *bioidentical*. Therefore, even though some hormones are produced in a laboratory, they are still called natural and bioidentical if they match the chemical structure in your body. Anything else is called synthetic.

The government-sponsored Women's Health Initiative program halted its study on estrogen plus progestin (synthetic progesterone, or Prempro) on July 9, 2002. The study was conducted on 16,000 women who had not had a hysterectomy. Participants were either given Prempro or a placebo. The study was ended three years earlier than initially planned because researchers found that there was an increased risk of breast cancer in some of the women who were participating in the trial and taking the hormones. In addition, synthetic hormones also give incomplete messages, and they do not balance the other hormones your own body produces.

The results of the Women's Health Initiative study brought to the forefront the reason why synthetic hormonal therapy will become a treatment of the past. A groundbreaking article by Dr. Kent Holtorf was published in the medical journal *Postgraduate Medicine* in January 2009. Dr. Holtorf's article answered the question of whether natural hormones are safer or more efficacious than synthetic hormones. After an extensive review of medical literature, the article concluded that the "physiological data and clinical outcomes demonstrate that bioidentical hormones are associated with lower risks, including the risk of breast cancer and cardiovascular disease, and are more efficacious than their synthetic and animal-derived counterparts. Until evidence is found to the contrary, bioidentical hormones remain the preferred method of HRT."

Bioidentical HRT (BHRT)

The results of the Women's Health Initiative study highlight the problems associated with "one size fits all" hormone replacement, which is when all women suffering hormonal problems—regardless of their symptoms—are instructed to take the same type and dosage of hormones. What is needed is for doctors and other healthcare providers to more carefully evaluate each woman's own unique set of environmental, genetic, and physiological risk factors to develop an HRT plan that is designed to fit her individual needs. For this, there is natural hormone replacement.

If you are taking natural hormone replacement, it means you are using hormones that are biologically identical to, or the same chemical structure as, the ones your body makes. One size does *not* fit all in medicine today; it is all about a customized approach to health care, otherwise known as *Personalized Medicine.* Studies have shown that BHRT does not increase your risk of developing breast cancer; in fact, it lowers your risks if you are given doses that are similar to what your own body makes.

---

breast cancer incidence with cancers more commonly node-positive. Moreover, breast cancer mortality also appears to be increased with combined estrogen plus progestin use.

POSSIBLE SIDE EFFECTS OF PROGESTINS

Progestins may have other side effects that do not occur with bioidentical progesterone.

- Acne
- Bloating
- Breakthrough bleeding/spotting
- Breast tenderness
- Counteracts many of the positive effects estrogen has on serotonin
- Decrease in energy
- Decrease in sexual interest
- Decreased HDL (good cholesterol)
- Depression
- Fluid retention
- Hair loss
- Headaches
- Inability to help produce estrogen and testosterone
- Increased appetite
- Increased LDL (bad cholesterol)
- Insomnia

- Irritability

- Nausea

- Protects only the uterus from cancer (not the breasts)

- Rashes

- Weight gain

- Remains in your body longer than bioidentical progesterone or prescribed bioidentical progesterone, which can prevent it from balancing with other hormones

- Spasms of the coronary arteries

Bioidentical progesterone offers a safer approach to HRT than synthetic progesterone (progestin) does. It is also very important that you have your levels of progesterone measured before you begin HRT, and then on a regular basis afterwards to confirm that you are taking an optimal dose for you. (See the section on testing on page 111.)

Progesterone can be used orally (by mouth) or transdermally (on the skin). If you're suffering from insomnia and you need to take progesterone, you should opt for the pill form. The pill affects the gamma-aminobutyric acid (GABA) receptors in your brain. GABA is an amino acid that acts as a neurotransmitter. It has a calming effect on your brain, which helps you sleep.

Bioidentical progesterone is also available as Prometrium, which is a pill derived from peanut oil made by a pharmaceutical company. The absorption rate of oral progesterone may change over the years, so you need less medication as you grow older. As women age, progesterone orally is most often used. Some women experience side effects from oral progesterone, such as nausea, breast swelling, dizziness, drowsiness, and depression, due to its effects on the liver and gastrointestinal tract. If you develop any of these symptoms, you should contact your healthcare provider to have your hormone levels measured and, if needed, a gut-health test done to determine if your GI tract is functioning optimally.

Many women who have had a complete hysterectomy wonder if they still need progesterone. The answer is categorically yes. Bioidentical progesterone has many positive effects on the body, as previously discussed.

Lastly, adrenaline also interacts with progesterone. When a person feels stressed, adrenaline surges, which can block progesterone receptors. This can prevent progesterone from being used effectively by the body.

THERAPEUTIC BENEFITS OF PROGESTERONE

The benefits of progesterone are many. Progesterone is a wonderful anti-flammatory agent and balances estrogen so that it decreases your risk of developing breast cancer. It also helps with anxiety, irritability, insomnia, mood swings, depression, heart racing, bladder problems, and gut disturbances along with having many other wonderful therapeutic benefits.

Estrogen/Progesterone Ratio

You've already learned about estrogen and progesterone. But did you know that it is important that the two hormones remain locked in a specific ratio within your body? The increase in inflammatory agents in today's world are enhancing estrogen levels (or estrogen-like chemicals) and estrogen dominance, which has increased greatly over the years.

As you will discover, there is an increased risk of breast cancer if estrogen metabolism favors the 16-hydroxyestrone pathway or the 4-hydroxyestrone pathway. There is also a higher risk for breast cancer if you have a low progesterone-to-estrogen ratio, meaning that the estrogen and progesterone ratio in your body is out of balance. Having a low progesterone-to-estrogen ratio can have other effects on the body, as well.

Effects of a Low Progesterone-to-Estrogen Ratio

- Abnormal bleeding during peri- and postmenopause
- Increase in some autoimmune diseases
- Increased risk of breast cancer
- Increased risk of uterine cancer
- Infertility

Estrogen and progesterone work together in your body. E2 (one of the forms of estrogen your body makes) lowers body fat by decreasing the amount of lipoprotein lipase, an enzyme, in your fat cells. Progesterone increases body fat storage by increasing the amount of lipoprotein lipase.

Estrogen and progesterone also work in concert to balance your body's release of insulin. E2 increases insulin sensitivity and improves glucose tolerance. Progesterone decreases insulin sensitivity and can cause insulin resistance. For this reason, women who have diabetes need to make sure that their estrogen/progesterone ratio is normal.

You *can* have too much of a good thing! If you have elevated levels of progesterone in relationship to estrogen, you can have many of the same side effects of having low progesterone. Also, if you use progesterone for too long without adequate estrogen, there can be negative effects on the body from decreased libido to weight gain to insulin resistance, to name a few.

When you have a salivary test or blood spot test done to measure your hormone levels, your healthcare practitioner or pharmacist will also receive a measure of the estrogen/progesterone ratio. Your healthcare provider will then prescribe the appropriate treatment, according to the lab results.

TESTOSTERONE

Testosterone falls into a class of hormones called *androgen*. Androgens are commonly referred to as "male" hormones, but they are present in women as well. For women, testosterone is made in the ovaries with a small amount produced in the adrenal glands. For most women as they age, the ovaries produce less testosterone. Women who have increased levels of androgens have higher levels of free testosterone. Therefore, it is important for women to measure their salivary levels and not just their total testosterone blood hormone levels, since saliva testing measures the free form of testosterone.

FUNCTIONS OF TESTOSTERONE IN YOUR BODY

Testosterone performs many important functions in the body.

- Aids in pain control
- Decreases bone deterioration
- Decreases excess body fat
- Elevates norepinephrine in the brain (has the same effect as taking an antidepressant)
- Helps maintain memory
- Increases muscle mass and strength
- Increases muscle tone (so your skin doesn't sag)
- Increases sense of emotional well-being, self-confidence, and motivation
- Increases sexual interest (86 percent of woman say they experience a decrease in sexual interest with menopause)

Women of any age can experience a deficiency of testosterone, which is indicated by a variety of symptoms. This hormone can be replaced transdermally (on the skin) if the levels are low.

Like other hormones, you can have too much testosterone in your body. Excess production of androgens is usually due to overproduction by your adrenal glands, but this can also be from your ovaries. Androgen dominance is the most common hormonal disorder in women. Many women have had or will have a form of androgen imbalance in their lifetime.

In younger women, adrenal imbalance is commonly related to PCOS. As women go through menopause, about 20 percent of them will experience high testosterone levels that will not decline with age. It is vitally important to work with your healthcare provider to lower this level, since the signs and symptoms of excess testosterone are many. High levels of testosterone increase your risk of developing breast cancer and also increase your risk of developing insulin resistance.

CAUSES OF ELEVATED TESTOSTERONE LEVELS

- Aggressive exercise program

- High DHEA levels, which may raise testosterone

- Perimenopause/menopause

- Polycystic ovarian syndrome (PCOS)

- Prescribed a dose of testosterone that is too high

WAYS TO LOWER TESTOSTERONE LEVELS

- *Camellia sinensis* (green tea): 270 mg works by increases SHBG

- *Glycyrrhiza glabra* (licorice root): 3.5 g licorice containing 7.6 percent glycyrrhizic acid decreases testosterone synthesis

- Saw palmetto: 240–260 mg twice a day

- Spearmint tea lowers testosterone levels and may raise FSH and LH

- Spironolactone: 100 mg twice a day. This is the least favorite of these methods. (It is a prescription and may have side effects, so other methods are suggested first)

- *Urtica dioica* (nettle): 300 mg twice a day. The root binds to and increases SHBG, which decreases the amount of bioavailable testosterone

- White peony (*Paeonia lactiflora*) increases progesterone, reduces elevated testosterone, modulates estrogen, and modulates prolactin

Any attempt to reduce testosterone levels should be made under the guidance of a healthcare professional. If none of the above-referenced methods are successful, then discuss the matter with your healthcare provider further. Metformin is a medication that is used to lower blood sugar, but it can also lower testosterone in the body. (See page 146 for more information on Metformin.) Depending on your personal health care needs, your doctor may prescribe this treatment.

TESTOSTERONE AND ESTROGEN

Research shows that for testosterone to work optimally, E2 must also be optimized. Without enough estrogen present, testosterone cannot attach to your brain receptors. Therefore, estrogen plays a role in how well testosterone works in your body.

If testosterone is taken with E2, it lowers your cardiac risk. If your estrogen levels are low and you take testosterone alone, it can increase plaque formation in the vessels of your heart, which increases your risk of developing heart disease.

Natural testosterone is the preferred method of testosterone replacement. Synthetic testosterone, or methyltestosterone, has been associated with an increased risk of liver cancer. Natural testosterone is effective when taken as a pill or applied as a cream, but it is much more commonly used as a cream. However, if you are using it as a cream, remember to rotate application sites. Applying the cream to the same location all the time will result in an increase in hair growth in that area. Testosterone replacement helps with aging skin, anxiety, and improves memory and decreases the risk of bone loss. It also aids weight loss.

DHEA

DHEA (*dehydroepiandrosterone*) is another sex hormone. It is made by your adrenal glands, but a small amount is also made in your brain and skin. DHEA is also converted into estrogen and testosterone.

DHEA production declines with age, starting in the late twenties. By the age of seventy, your body makes only one-fourth of the amount it made earlier. Furthermore, DHEA levels change if you are stressed long-term. When you begin to experience stress, DHEA levels can initially increase. Overtime, if you remain stressed, DHEA levels start to drop and can become too low in the body. Low DHEA levels can occur at any age.

FUNCTIONS OF DHEA

DHEA has many functions in the body from helping you maintain bone structure, memory maintenance, to supporting your immune system to helping you deal with stress. It also acts as an anti-inflammatory and reduces your blood sugar.

SIGNS AND SYMPTOMS OF DHEA DEFICIENCY

☐ Decreased energy

☐ Decreased muscle strength and lean body mass

☐ Difficulty in dealing with stress

☐ Increased risk of infection

☐ Insomnia

☐ Insulin resistance

☐ Irritability

☐ Joint soreness

☐ Osteopenia/osteoporosis

☐ Weight gain

There are many things that can contribute to DHEA deficiency. If your body has a low DHEA level, it would be a good idea to consider DHEA replacement. There are many benefits of replacing DHEA, which can be supplemented orally or as a cream. For example, DHEA has been shown to have a protective effect against cancer, diabetes, obesity, high cholesterol, heart disease, and some autoimmune diseases.

In studies conducted at the University of Tennessee, supplementation with DHEA produced a 30 percent reduction in insulin levels when compared to taking the diabetes drug metformin alone. Importantly, the supplements also tripled patients' sensitivity to insulin. This result may be related to the idea that diabetics may have lower levels of DHEA in their bodies than people who have normal blood sugar levels.

In the elderly, DHEA helps increase the immune system ability to fight infections. DHEA also improves physical and psychological well-being, muscle strength, and bone density, and reduces body fat and age-related skin atrophy, stimulating procollagen/sebum production. Moreover, DHEA controls cardiovascular-signaling pathways and exerts anti-inflammatory, and widen blood vessels. Therefore, low levels of DHEA correlate with increased cardiovascular disease and death due to all causes.

In addition, DHEA appears to be protective against asthma and allergies by attenuating allergic inflammation and reducing eosinophilia and airway hyperreactivity. Eosinophilia refers to a high eosinophil (a kind of white blood cell) count that occurs with infection or allergy. Furthermore, in women, DHEA improves sexual satisfaction, fertility, and age-related vaginal atrophy (thinning, drying, and inflammation of the vaginal walls).

However, like most other hormones, you can have too much DHEA in your body which can cause any number of symptoms. If you have had hormonal related breast cancer (ER+ and/or PR+) then you should never replace DHEA.

CORTISOL

Cortisol is one of only two hormones in your body that increases with age. It is also one of your sex hormones. Like DHEA, cortisol is made by your adrenal glands, which make all your sex hormones after menopause. Cortisol levels are regulated by the *adrenocorticotropic hormone* (ACTH), which is produced by the pituitary gland. Cortisol is commonly known as the "stress hormone," due to its involvement in your response to stress.

- Low levels of cortisol are characterized as hypocortisolism, hypoadrenalism, or adrenal fatigue.

- High levels of cortisol are characterized as hypercortisolism or hyperadrenalism.

- When no cortisol is produced, Addison's disease is indicated.

- When extremely high levels of cortisol are produced, Cushing's disease is indicated.

Stressful life events trigger psychological processes that can affect health behaviors and hormone balance regulation through the following pathways, which may then increase your risk of developing breast cancer and/or a reoccurrence.

- Stressors can adversely affect one's psychological well-being.

- The negative emotional responses that occur with stress can cause an imbalance in biochemistry and physiology in the body and can contribute to this disease.

- When someone is stressed, they commonly increase risky behaviors (such as eating a lot of sugar and smoking) that increases your risk of developing breast cancer and a reoccurrence.

- Individuals that are stressed commonly do not see their healthcare provider as often.

In fact, studies have revealed the physiological effects of cortisol on mammary gland development, estrogen activity, and other intracellular pathways involved in breast cancer development. Scientific evidence has strengthened the premise that stressful life events can lead to an increased chance of developing breast cancer and a reoccurrence.

FUNCTIONS OF CORTISOL IN YOUR BODY

- Acts as an anti-inflammatory
- Affects pituitary/thyroid/adrenal system
- Balances blood sugar
- Balances DHEA
- Controls weight
- Improves mood and thoughts
- Influences estrogen/testosterone ratio
- Participates with aldosterone in sodium reabsorption
- Promotes good sleep hygiene
- Regulates bone turnover rate
- Regulates immune system response
- Regulates the stress reaction
- Supports protein synthesis

CONDITIONS ASSOCIATED WITH ABNORMAL LEVELS OF CORTISOL

Abnormal cortisol levels that are too high or too low can be associated with many medical conditions.

- Alzheimer's disease
- Anorexia nervosa
- Breast cancer
- Chronic fatigue syndrome
- Coronary heart disease
- Depression
- Diabetes
- Exacerbations of multiple sclerosis
- Fibromyalgia
- Generalized memory loss
- Heart disease
- Impotence
- Infertility
- Insulin resistance
- Irritable bowel syndrome (IBS)
- Menopause
- Osteoporosis
- Panic disorders
- PMS
- Post-traumatic stress disorder (PTSD)
- Rheumatoid arthritis
- Sleep disorders
- Weight gain

There is a strong interrelationship between activation of the *hypothalamic-pituitary-adrenal* (HPA) axis and energy balance. Individuals with abdominal obesity tend to have elevated cortisol levels. Furthermore, stress and cortisol act to control both food intake and energy expenditure. Cortisol is known to increase the consumption of foods high in fat and sugar in animals and humans. In women, high-cortisol individuals eat more in response to stress than low-cortisol, leading to increased food intake and reduced energy expenditure, and thus a predisposition to obesity. Therefore, cortisol responsiveness may be used as a marker to identify people who are at risk of weight gain and subsequent obesity.

The optimal method of measuring cortisol for the purpose of balancing your hormones is salivary testing. An assay for cortisol levels will not be accurate if you have been on steroids within the last thirty days. Contact your healthcare provider to discuss steroid use and cortisol measurement if you are taking prescription steroids. If you require long-term steroid treatment for another medical problem, your doctor can take this information into account when interpreting the results of the saliva test. If you are on steroids short-term, then usually your healthcare provider will not have you do saliva testing within one month of your using a prescription for a steroid medication (such as an asthma inhaler).

When you are stressed, your cortisol levels increase. When you are stressed for a long time, then your cortisol levels can become too low. Your body requires cortisol, however, to survive. Therefore, when cortisol becomes too low, your adrenal gland will convert pregnenolone hormone into cortisol, no matter what age you are, even if it means depleting your body of pregnenolone.

When your adrenal glands do not produce enough cortisol, this can lead to serious health issues and become life-threatening. Symptoms can include extreme fatigue, low blood pressure, loss of appetite, weight loss, and stress issues. When cortisol and DHEA levels drop, your body goes into a state of adrenal fatigue called hypoadrenalism. Adrenal fatigue is not a total depletion of cortisol, but it does bring cortisol levels down low enough to prevent optimal functioning of the body. Adrenal fatigue is one of the most pervasive and underdiagnosed syndromes of modern society.

If the adrenals become totally depleted, this condition is called Addison's disease. If you have Addison's disease, your body makes no cortisol at all. A deficiency of cortisol that is not Addison's disease is usually caused by stress.

SIGNS AND SYMPTOMS OF ADRENAL FATIGUE (CORTISOL DEFICIENCY)

☐ Allergies (environmental sensitivities and chemical intolerance)

☐ Decreased immunity

☐ Decreased sexual interest

- [ ] Digestive problems
- [ ] Drug addiction
- [ ] Emotional imbalances
- [ ] Emotional paralysis
- [ ] Fatigue
- [ ] Feeling overwhelmed
- [ ] General feeling of "unwellness"
- [ ] Hypoglycemia (low blood sugar)
- [ ] Increased PMS, perimenopausal, and menopausal symptoms

- [ ] Increased risk of alcoholism and drug addiction
- [ ] Lack of stamina
- [ ] Loss of motivation or initiative
- [ ] Low blood pressure
- [ ] Poor healing of wounds
- [ ] Progressively poorer athletic performance
- [ ] Sensitivity to light
- [ ] Unresponsive hypothyroidism (low thyroid function that doesn't respond to treatment)

CAUSES OF LOW CORTISOL

- Chronic inflammation
- Chronic pain
- Depression
- Dysbiosis
- Hypoglycemia
- Long-term stress
- Nutritional deficiencies
- Overly aggressive exercise
- Poor sleep
- Severe allergies
- Toxic exposure

If your cortisol level is too low due to adrenal fatigue from long-term stress, begin your therapy with stress reduction techniques. Your doctor will also start you on a multivitamin. Your adrenal glands need vitamin C, B vitamins, calcium, magnesium, zinc, selenium, copper, sodium, and manganese. Adaptogenic herbs are also very beneficial, such as ashwagandha, *Panax ginseng*, *Rhodiola rosea*, and *Cordyceps sinensis*. Calming herbs such as chamomile and lemon balm can be very beneficial. If you are not improving, your healthcare provider may discontinue the adaptogenic herbs and begin you on adrenal extracts after approximately six months.

If your cortisol level is still low after another three to six months, then your doctor may add licorice root to your therapy regimen. Licorice root decreases the amount of hydrocortisone that is broken down by the liver, which reduces the demand on the adrenals to produce more cortisol. Licorice root can raise your blood pressure, so it should not be taken if you have hypertension. If you develop high blood pressure while taking it, then discontinue its use.

If your DHEA level is low, your healthcare provider can prescribe you DHEA if you have not had hormonal related breast cancer. It is important that you also take herbal therapies, otherwise when your DHEA is measured again the level may be even lower despite your taking it. If all other therapies fail and your cortisol level is still low, then your healthcare provider may prescribe Cortef to take for six months. It is the therapy of last resort. Your doctor will keep you on adrenal extract or adaptogenic herbs while you are taking Cortef so that you have a therapy available for your body to use when it comes time to wean yourself off Cortef, which can take at least a month.

Usually, it takes six months of constant stress or more for adrenal fatigue to settle in. However, once you start treatment for your exhausted adrenals, it takes one to two years for your glands to heal completely.

There are other things you can do to help treat adrenal fatigue. Restful sleep (sleeping until 9 am or later), resolving a stressful situation, lying down during a break from work, going to bed early (around 9 pm), and avoiding eating fruit in the morning can all help. Clearly, trying these options before things get out of hand is a good idea. If adrenal fatigue can be helped or improved, the overall healing time will be shortened.

Many women who have adrenal fatigue also have a thyroid that isn't functioning to its full potential (hypothyroidism). It is important to always work on fixing the adrenal glands before thyroid medication is instituted; otherwise, the symptoms of adrenal fatigue may be made worse.

Adrenal fatigue is a symptom that can dramatically affect your health and can be reversed with proper treatment. Lifestyle changes, good nutrition, dietary supplements, and stress reduction techniques have all proven to be effective.

CORTISOL AND STRESS

When you are stressed, cortisol levels rise. As stress decreases, levels come back down. However, in today's world, a lot of people are stressed a lot of the time. Overbooking is an issue for almost everyone. If you have too many tasks on your plate or you multitask all the time, your body will remain in a state of constant stress. One study showed that as many as 75 percent to 90 percent of visits to primary care doctors are related to stress. In fact, chronic stress has been shown to contribute to accelerated aging and premature death. Another study revealed that chronic stress accelerated the aging process and was associated with shortened telomeres.

The most important thing you can do to get rid of your stress is to gain control of your time. Learn to say "no" kindly. Know how much work and responsibility you can take on without feeling overwhelmed, and do not take on more than you can handle. It is also useful to practice some relaxing techniques that you can turn to in times of stress. Running a hot bath, drinking a cup of coffee or tea, listening to your favorite song, or curling up with a good book are all effective ways to reduce stress. Figure out what works for you and turn to it if you feel your stress levels rising.

Stress can be harnessed to fuel success and achievement. However, if your stress is to the point of "distress," then that is a problem. Magnesium, potassium, B vitamins, vitamin C, zinc, carbohydrates, and other nutrients are used up when you are stressed.

Your brain is one of the body parts that is most affected by stress. When you are stressed and your cortisol levels increase, your body produces more free radicals. This damages your neurons and decreases your ability to think and remember things. When this happens, your body's ability to change short-term memories into long-term memories is affected. Your ability to recall and retrieve information is also impacted by stress. High levels of cortisol are associated with deterioration of the hippocampus, the part of your brain that processes memory.

Other Signs of Stress

By this point, you have learned that stress greatly affects cortisol levels, causing them to elevate. Elevated cortisol levels can have many negative consequences. (See page 138.) Over the years, I have compiled a list of common signs of stress, which can be divided into four categories.

Behavioral symptoms may be seen in the way you act. Some behavioral symptoms include bossiness, compulsive eating or gum chewing, excessive smoking, grinding your teeth at night, alcohol abuse, and an inability to focus on and complete tasks.

Cognitive symptoms are those that affect the way you think. If you are stressed, you may experience constant worry, forgetfulness, memory loss, or a lack of creativity. Additionally, you may have difficulty making decisions, lose your sense of humor, or have thoughts of running away.

Emotional symptoms affect your mood and feelings. If you're stressed, you may find that you are easily upset. Additionally, you may experience a range of emotions, including anger, boredom, edginess, loneliness, nervousness, anxiety, and unhappiness. Finally, people who are stressed commonly feel like they are under pressure, and they often feel powerless to change anything.

Lastly, there are some physical symptoms of stress that can affect your body. These include back pain, dizziness, headaches, a racing heart, restlessness, indigestion, stomachaches, tiredness, sweaty palms, a stiff neck or shoulders, ringing in the ears, and difficulty sleeping.

If you find that you are experiencing any of these symptoms, it would be a good idea to try and lower your levels of stress. (Some suggestions for how you can do this are on pages 136–137.) You will greatly benefit in the long run.

In addition to stress, cortisol levels also increase with depression, high progestin intake, use of birth control pills, infections, inadequate sleep, inflammation, hypoglycemia (low blood sugar), toxic exposure, pain, and toxic exposure.

SIGNS AND SYMPTOMS OF ELEVATED CORTISOL

☐ Binge eating

☐ Compromised immune system

☐ Confusion

☐ Fatigue

☐ Favors the development of leaky gut syndrome

☐ Impaired hepatic conversion of T4 to T3 (see thyroid section on page 154)

☐ Increased blood pressure

☐ Increased blood sugar

☐ Increased cholesterol

☐ Increased insulin and insulin resistance

☐ Increased risk of developing osteoporosis/osteopenia

☐ Increased susceptibility to bruise

☐ Increased susceptibility to infections

☐ Increased triglycerides

☐ Irritability

☐ Low energy

☐ Night sweats

☐ Shakiness between meals

☐ Sleep disturbances

☐ Sugar cravings

☐ Thinning skin

☐ Weakened muscles

Lowering your cortisol level, if it is elevated, is very important. Stress-reduction techniques and a multivitamin are key components to start you on your way to normalizing your cortisol level. Adaptogenic herbs such as ashwagandha, *Panax ginseng, Rhodiola rosea, Cordyceps sinensis, Ginkgo biloba,* and others are very beneficial if you feel stressed, and calming herbs such as lemon balm and chamomile are helpful if you feel wired. If cortisol is high in the evening, then add phosphatidylserine (300 mg) which may be taken at any point during the day. Long-term elevated levels of cortisol in the evening increase your risk of developing breast cancer and a reoccurrence.

SUMMARY

Optimal cortisol levels help prevent many disease processes, in fact, almost all diseases including breast cancer. A small amount of stress helps your body heal. Too much stress harms your body. Stress reduction techniques are a key component to healing. Prayer, meditation, tai chi (a Chinese form of martial arts), yoga, chi gong (a form of body and mind therapy), breathing exercises and techniques, exercise (not strenuous exercise if you have adrenal fatigue), music, acupuncture, and dancing have all been shown to be therapeutic.

To be healthy, you must be physically healthy, emotionally healthy, and spiritually healthy. All these areas of your life must be optimally functioning in order for you to enjoy a stress-free existence. If you stay stressed long-term it compromises not just your overall health but increases your risk of developing breast cancer, and if you have had the disease increases your chance of getting it again.

INSULIN

Insulin is the hormone responsible for the regulation of blood sugar. It is produced in the pancreas. Insulin affects the balance of other hormones as other hormones affect the balance of insulin. Perfect insulin levels are a key to the best health possible. Insulin levels that are too high or too low can cause symptoms and increase the risk of developing several diseases such as diabetes and breast cancer.

As you have seen in previous chapters, blood sugar regulation is related to several other controllable risk factors for breast cancer. This includes diet, sugar, high fructose corn syrup, and obesity.

FUNCTIONS OF INSULIN

- Aids other nutrients to get inside cells

- Counters the actions of adrenaline and cortisol in the body

- Has an anti-inflammatory effect on endothelial cells and macrophages

- Helps convert blood sugar into triglycerides

- Helps the body repair itself

- Increases expression of some lipogenic enzymes

- Keeps blood glucose levels from rising too high

- Partially regulates protein turnover rate

- Plays a major role in the production of serotonin

- Stimulates the development of muscle (but at high levels it turns off the production of muscle and increases the production of fat)

- Suppresses reactive oxygen species (ROS)

Have your healthcare provider measure your fasting insulin level. Fasting serum insulin is used as an index of insulin sensitivity and resistance. The optimal fasting insulin level is 6 uIU/mL. Insulin levels that are too low or too high indicate that our insulin is not working optimally in your body. Commonly your doctor will measure your fasting blood sugar (FBS) and maybe also your hemoglobin A1c. Your hemoglobin A1c test tells you your average level of blood sugar over the past two to three months. It is rare unless you see a practitioner who specializes in Personalized Medicine that you would have your fasting insulin level measured. To make sure your fasting insulin level is in balance, consider requesting this test from your doctor.

SIGNS AND SYMPTOMS OF INSULIN DEFICIENCY

☐ Blurred vision

☐ Bone loss

☐ Confusion

☐ Depression

☐ Dizziness

☐ Fainting

☐ Fatigue

☐ Hunger

☐ Hypoglycemia

☐ Insomnia

☐ Insulin resistance

☐ Loss of consciousness (late-stage)

☐ Palpitations

☐ Seizures (late-stage)

☐ Sweating

CAUSES OF INSULIN DEFICIENCY

- Eliminating carbohydrates from the diet

- Hypopituitarism

- Insulin resistance/diabetes (See page 143.)

- Not eating enough

- Overexercising without sufficient food and nutritional support

- Pancreatic diseases such as chronic pancreatitis, cancer of the pancreas, and cystic fibrosis

When you eat complex carbohydrates and simple sugars, your insulin levels climb. If you eat too much sugar, your body produces more and more insulin until the insulin level is elevated and it does not work as effectively as it should. The medical term for this is *insulin resistance.*

Conditions Associated with Excess Insulin Production

- Accelerated aging
- Acne
- Acromegaly
- Asthma
- Breast Cancer
- Cushing's syndrome
- Depression
- Estrogen levels that are too low
- Heart disease
- Heartburn
- Hypercholesterolemia
- Hypertension
- Hypertriglyceridemia
- Increased risk of developing cancer
- Infertility
- Insomnia
- Insulin resistance/diabetes
- Irritable bowel syndrome
- Metabolic syndrome
- Migraine headaches
- Mood swings
- Osteopenia/osteoporosis
- Weight gain

Insulin is part of the hormonal symphony in your body, so when it is not performing optimally, all the other hormones are affected. Your body will attempt to compensate for insulin's decreased effects by producing more and more insulin. This can result in high insulin levels all the time, which can cause the cells in your adrenal glands, called theca cells, to turn on an enzyme called 17, 20-lyase. This enzyme causes your body's hormones to stop making estrogens and instead make androgens. (Both estrogens and androgens are made from DHEA.) This shift in hormonal balance can cause you to gain weight around the middle. It may also promote further insulin resistance. In fact, prolonged levels of high insulin can lead to diabetes. Furthermore, most major processes that lead to hardening of the arteries are caused by the overproduction of insulin.

When you eat simple sugars and consume caffeine to help with fatigue, not only will your cortisol level become abnormal, but this will contribute to an elevated level of insulin in your body. Additionally, this causes your body to produce gas, and you may experience bloating. Water is pulled into your colon from the bloodstream to respond to the high sugar load, which can lead to loose stools. You may develop gluten sensitivity from overeating carbohydrates.

There are many habits that can elevate insulin besides eating a diet high in simple sugars. Having a lot of stress, which causes your cortisol levels to be abnormal, will have a negative impact on insulin production. The following list contains lifestyle choices that raise insulin, as per Dr. Diana Schwarzbein, an endocrinologist and author of *The Schwarzbein Principle* and *The Schwarzbein Principle II.*

CAUSES OF EXCESS INSULIN PRODUCTION

- Cigarette smoking
- Consuming soft drinks
- Eating a low-fat diet
- Eating trans fats (partially hydrogenated or hydrogenated)
- Elevated DHEA levels
- Excessive alcohol consumption
- Excessive caffeine intake
- Excessive or unnecessary thyroid hormone replacement
- Excessive progesterone replacement
- Increased testosterone levels (male or female)
- Lack of exercise
- Poor sleep hygiene
- Skipping meals
- Some over-the-counter cold medications (any that contain caffeine)
- Some prescription medications
- Stress
- Taking diet pills
- Taking thyroid hormone replacement while not eating enough
- Use of artificial sweeteners
- Use of natural stimulants
- Use of recreational stimulants
- Yo-yo dieting

Elevated insulin levels can be lowered by eating a balanced diet of carbohydrates, proteins, and fats. The right amount of exercise (three or four times a week) can help to normalize insulin levels. Changing medications, quitting smoking, discontinuing stimulants, and decreasing or stopping caffeine consumption can also be beneficial. In addition, there are nutrients that can help insulin work more effectively in the body. Alpha-lipoic acid, chromium, and vitamin D all do just this. However, these supplements can be very powerful, so if you are already taking a drug that lowers your blood sugar, you may need less medication with the use of these products.

Make sure you monitor your blood sugar closely. Alpha-lipoic acid has even been shown to prevent and treat diabetic neuropathy, a condition in which the body's nerves become damaged due to diabetes. (See *Insulin Resistance* on page 143 for further information.)

THERAPEUTIC BENEFITS OF OPTIMAL INSULIN LEVELS

- Helps to normalize weight
- Memory maintenance
- Prevention and treatment of insulin resistance and diabetes
- Prevention and treatment of polycystic ovary syndrome (PCOS)
- Prevention of coronary heart disease
- Prevention of hypertension
- Prevention of osteoporosis/osteopenia
- Prevention of some cancers such as breast cancer

INSULIN RESISTANCE

Insulin resistance (IR) is evident when cells do not properly absorb glucose, the body's preferred source of fuel, resulting in a buildup of glucose in the blood. From a medical viewpoint, insulin resistance is defined as a reduced response to insulin stimulation in tissues such as the liver, muscle, and adipose tissue. This hinders the ability of the body to dispose of glucose and causes the body to produce excess amounts of insulin. This is called hyperinsulinemia. IR can be a result of obesity, but it can also be influenced by hereditary factors.

Increased estrogen levels caused by the aromatization of androgens in adipose tissue may increase breast tissue cell growth. Moreover, if left untreated, insulin resistance may lead to prediabetes, a condition in which glucose levels are higher than normal but not high enough to be considered diabetes. Insulin resistance occurs when insulin is present but does not work as effectively in the body as it should. Consequently, levels start to rise to help the body compensate for less than effective insulin function.

More than 80 percent of the adult population in the United States has blood glucose levels that are too high. If an individual has a fasting blood sugar (FBS) that is high-normal (over 85 mg/dL), the risk of the patient dying of cardiovascular disease (heart disease) is increased by 40 percent. Furthermore, having a FBS that is high-normal increases the risk of heart disease, stroke, diabetes, cognitive decline, obesity, and breast cancer.

SIGNS AND SYMPTOMS OF INSULIN RESISTANCE

☐ Fuzzy brain

☐ Infertility

☐ Irregular menstrual cycles

☐ Irritability

☐ Loose bowel movements, alternating with constipation

☐ Water retention

☐ Weight gain

CAUSES OF INSULIN RESISTANCE

Insulin resistance has many possible causes. Here are some reasons why individuals with insulin resistance are not able to effectively use insulin.

- Abuse of alcohol
- Decreased estrogen
- Eating processed foods
- Elevated DHEA levels
- Excessive caffeine intake
- Excessive dieting
- Excessive progesterone in females (prescribed)
- Genetic susceptibility
- Hypothyroidism
- Increased stress
- Increased testosterone
- Insomnia
- Lack of exercise
- Use of nicotine
- Use of oral contraceptives and other forms of progestin

INSULIN RESISTANCE AND BREAST CANCER

Insulin is a crucial growth agent that promotes cancer by boosting cell duplication and migration while also decreasing the death of cancerous cells. In one study, a total of 22,837 postmenopausal women found that higher levels of insulin resistance were associated with higher breast cancer incidence and death from any cause after the diagnosis of breast cancer.

Importantly, insulin resistance affects the development of breast cancer in three significant ways.

1. Insulin resistance leads to an increase in aromatase and a decrease in sex hormone binding, which increases the amount of estrogen that is unbound and available for the body to use. This then leads to activated P13K and Ras/MAPK/Akt pathways, which lead to the development of breast cancer cells through an increase in tumor epithelial cell growth, invasion, and spread. This then affects cell growth, migration, and invasion, which all affect survival rates.

2. Insulin resistance leads to elevated glucose levels (hyperglycemia) and hyperlipidemia (high triglyceride and elevated cholesterol) leads to metabolic reprogramming. This reprogramming leads to glucotoxicity, lipotoxicity (a metabolic syndrome that results from the accumulation of lipid intermediates in non-fat tissue, leading to cellular dysfunction and death), oxidative stress, and aberrant autophagy which leads to cellular damage which also affects survival rates.

3. Insulin resistance is associated with high leptin levels, low adiponectin levels (see the Obesity section in Chapter 7, "Controllable Health Disorder Risk Factors," page 162), and an increase in vascular endothelial growth factor (VEGF) which leads to vascular endothelial cells which leads to angiogenesis which affects survival rates.

THERAPIES FOR INSULIN RESISTANCE

Conventional therapies for insulin resistance involve exercise and a diet centered on consumption of foods with low glycemic index numbers. If an individual is overweight, then weight reduction is very beneficial. If these methods are not successful, then medications such as metformin may be added.

Personalized Medicine has many therapies to improve and sometimes even reverse insulin resistance. The first one is exercise. Lack of exercise is a risk factor for the development of insulin resistance and diabetes in susceptible individuals. Exercising four days a week for an hour a day has been shown to be beneficial. Eating foods that are low on the glycemic index (GI) is important. The GI ranks carbohydrate-containing foods on a scale from 0 to 100, according to the speed with which they enter the bloodstream and raise glucose levels. Foods high on the list increase blood sugar and cause insulin to rise.

One study showed that insulin secretion was lower in people who were on a low glycemic index program for only two weeks. The glycemic index is affected by the size of the particles into which the food breaks down. Therefore, the more processed the food or the longer it is cooked, the higher its glycemic index. The best carbohydrates that curb insulin are broccoli, lentils, and chickpeas. In addition, the fat content of a food influences its glycemic index ranking. Fat slows down sugar absorption and therefore lowers the glycemic index number.

The right balance of saturated to polyunsaturated to monounsaturated fats is important both for the prevention and treatment of insulin resistance and diabetes. Likewise, a high-fiber diet is crucial. Soluble fiber has been shown to lower insulin levels. Furthermore, getting enough protein in the diet decreases the absorption of sugars and consequently decreases your glycemic load. Weight loss has been proven to be helpful as well. Moreover, getting a good

Metformin

In the past decade, a series of publications reported that patients with type II diabetes who were treated with the oral biguanide metformin (an anti-hyperglycemic medication) had a lower incidence of cancer than did their counterparts taking other medications for diabetes mellitus, including insulin and sulfonylureas.

How does Metformin work in relation to cancer? It requires activation of AMP-activated protein kinase (AMPK) to elicit its antidiabetic effects. AMPK is a crucial cellular energy sensor. AMPK signaling prompts cells to produce energy at the expense of growth and motility, opposing the actions of insulin and growth factors. Increasing AMPK activity may thus prevent the proliferation and metastasis of tumor cells. Activated AMPK also suppresses aromatase, which lowers estrogen formation and prevents breast cancer growth. Moreover, AMPK-dependent inhibition of insulin-stimulated growth has been demonstrated in several breast cancer cell lines. Metformin-induced AMPK activation in these cell lines led to growth inhibition (blockage).

Furthermore, emerging data have demonstrated that metformin can selectively kill cancer stem cells. Cancer stem cells (CSC) are a distinct subpopulation within a tumor. They can self-renew and differentiate and possess a high capability to repair DNA damage, exhibit low levels of reactive oxygen species (ROS), and proliferate (increase in numbers) slowly. These features render CSC resistant to various therapies, including radiation therapy. Therefore, elimination of all cancer stem cells is a requirement for effective therapy against all cancers including breast cancer. Consequently, CSC are the prime targets for any form of treatment.

Metformin is highly active against cancer growth, and clinical trials are currently being conducted for several different malignancies including breast cancer.

night's sleep has been shown to be beneficial. If you do not sleep at least six and a half hours a night, then insulin levels may rise and lead to insulin resistance.

There are also many nutritional supplements and botanical nutrients that have clinical trials supporting their use in insulin resistance.

SUMMARY

Many people in the United States and the remainder of the world have insulin resistance. The great news is that there are many therapies with proven clinical trials that have been shown to be beneficial in helping insulin to work more effectively in your body which will decrease your risk of developing breast cancer as well as a reoccurrence.

SUPPLEMENTS TO TREAT INSULIN RESISTANCE

Before starting any nutrients, discuss their use with your healthcare provider if you have a history of breast cancer.

Supplements	Dosage	Considerations
Alpha-lipoic acid	100 mg to 400 mg daily	Alpha-lipoic acid improves blood sugar levels, so diabetics may be able to take less medication. Alpha-lipoic acid also slows the development of diabetic neuropathy. Consult your healthcare provider if you are considering taking more than 500 mg in a day. Larger doses can negatively impact thyroid functioning.
Arginine	1,000 to 5,000 mg once a day	Do not take it if you have kidney disease, liver disease, or herpes except under a doctor's supervision. Arginine can interact with some medications. Consult with your healthcare provider before beginning this therapy.
B-complex vitamins	50 mg twice a day	I suggest taking a multivitamin along with your B-complex vitamins.
Berberine*	Start with 200 mg twice a day (you may go up to 500 mg three times a day)	Do not use this supplement during pregnancy. It can cause uterine contractions.
Bergamot	800 mg once or twice a day	It also blocks the rate-limiting step in cholesterol production. If you are on a cholesterol lowering medication, have your healthcare provider measure your cholesterol after three months. You may need a lower dose of the drug.
Carnitine*	2,000 to 3,000 mg once a day	Have your healthcare provider measure your TMAO levels before starting long-term supplementation with carnitine.
Carnosine	2,000 mg once a day	Check with your doctor before starting carnosine therapy if you have diabetes, hypertension, kidney disease, or liver damage. Too much carnosine can result in hyperactivity.
Chromium	300 to 1,000 mcg once a day as chromium picolinate	Combining with the protein picolinate allows your body to absorb chromium more efficiently. However, some chromium picolinate supplements contain more chromium than necessary. Ask your healthcare provider for a recommendation on chromium consumption.
Coenzyme Q_{10}*	30 to 200 mg daily	If you are on blood-thinning medications, speak to your healthcare provider before using CoQ_{10}. Since some medications can cause a deficiency of this nutrient, speak to your healthcare provider to determine if you might need a larger dose.
Cysteine	500 mg once a day as n-acetylcysteine, or NAC	When taking NAC supplements, also take extra vitamin C, copper, and zinc.
EPA/DHA (fish oil)*	1,000 to 2,000 mg once a day	Choose a source that contains vitamin E to prevent oxidation.

Fenugreek*	50 mg of seed powder twice a day, or 2 to 4.5 ml of 1:2 liquid extract twice a day	Avoid fenugreek if you are allergic to chickpeas, peanuts, green peas, or soybeans. Fenugreek has mild blood-thinning effects. If you have a bleeding disorder or are taking a medication or supplement that may thin your blood, do not take this herb. Fenugreek may also negatively impact thyroid functioning.
Fiber, soluble	Suggested daily intake is 25 grams for women and 38 grams for men (Try to get most of your fiber from whole foods)	Choose a fiber supplement with no added sugar and take it with several glasses of water to prevent side effects.
Ginkgo biloba*	120 mg once daily	Do not use with blood-thinning medications or supplements.
Green coffee bean extract	400 mg a day	Because green coffee contains caffeine, you should avoid taking this supplement if you are sensitive to caffeine.
Gymnema sylvestre	400 to 600 mg a day of an extract that contains 24 percent gymnemic acid	Stop taking this supplement two weeks before surgery, as it can interfere with blood sugar control during and after surgical procedures. At high doses, gymnema can cause gastric irritation or liver toxicity.
Inositol	2,000 to 4,000 mg once a day	May stimulate uterine contractions. Women who wish to become pregnant should consult their doctor regarding its use. Doses larger than 200 mg should be taken only under physician supervision.
Magnesium	400 to 800 mg once a day	Consult your healthcare provider for dosage if you have kidney disease. Discontinue use and see your doctor if you experience abdominal pain. Take a lower dose if it causes diarrhea.
Manganese	2 to 5 mg once a day	Use with caution if you have gallbladder or liver disease.
Olive leaf extract*	500 mg to 750 mg a day containing 20 mg of oleuropein per capsule	Olive leaf extracts can interact with many prescription medications and may increase the effects of blood thinners. Consult your healthcare provider before using olive leaf extract if you are taking any medication. Don't use it if you are pregnant or breastfeeding.
Selenium	200 mcg once a day	Do not exceed 200 mcg a day without consulting your healthcare provider.
Taurine	1,000 to 1,500 mg once a day	Take between meals. Discontinue use if you suddenly have feelings of chest or throat tightness or if you break out in hives. Do not take with aspirin. Have your healthcare provider measure levels before starting taurine therapy.
Vitamin D$_3$	Have your blood levels measured by your healthcare provider, who will determine proper dosage	You can become vitamin D toxic. Therefore, have your healthcare provider measure your levels to determine the perfect dose for you.

Zinc	20 to 50 mg once a day as zinc picolinate or zinc citrate	Your copper-to-zinc ratio is very important to your health. If you are taking zinc and iron supplements, take one in the morning and one in the evening. (Taking them together reduces the efficiency of both.)

*This supplement can have blood-thinning action.

MELATONIN

Melatonin is a hormone produced in the pineal gland, retina, GI tract, and white blood cells, and is associated with sleep. In addition, there are melatonin receptors expressed all over the body—for example, in the intestines, fat tissue, kidneys, liver, lungs, adrenals, and other organs. The amount of melatonin the body produces decreases as one ages and depends on the activity of an enzyme called serotonin-N-acetyltransferase (NAT). The body's production of NAT, on the other hand, depends on its storage of vitamin B_6. Melatonin has many functions in your body from building your immune system to being a therapy for breast cancer.

FUNCTIONS OF MELATONIN

- Acts as an antioxidant
- Aids the immune system
- Blocks estrogen from binding to receptor sites
- Decreases cortisol levels that are elevated
- Decreases platelet stickiness (decreases the risk of heart disease)
- Dilates and contracts blood vessels
- Effects the release of sex hormones
- Helps balance the stress response
- Helps prevent cancer and treat some cancers
- Improves mood
- Improves sleep quality
- Inhibits the release of insulin from beta cells in the pancreas
- Inhibits the release of prolactin, follicle stimulating hormone (FSH) and luteinizing hormone (LH)
- Is cardioprotective
- Promotes healthy cholesterol levels
- Protects against GI reflux
- Protects skin cells against UV damage
- Regulates skin pigmentation
- Relieves jet lag
- Stimulates the parathyroid gland
- Stimulates the production of growth hormone

SIGNS AND SYMPTOMS OF MELATONIN DEFICIENCY

☐ Anxiety

☐ Compromised immune system

☐ Early morning awakening

☐ Fatigue

☐ Heart disease

☐ Immunological disorders

☐ Increased risk of cancer

☐ Insomnia

☐ Interrupted sleep

☐ Seasonal affective disorder

☐ Stress

CAUSES OF MELATONIN DEFICIENCY

There are many reasons for melatonin deficiency. Perhaps the most common cause of melatonin deficiency in today's world is electromagnetic fields. This occurs in our everyday lives due to exposure to cell phone waves, Wi-Fi and Bluetooth waves, microwaves, radio broadcasting waves, and TV broadcasting waves. Other common causes are caffeine abuse, high glycemic index foods, tobacco, and some medications. B_{12} deficiency is also associated with low melatonin levels.

THERAPEUTIC BENEFITS OF MELATONIN

The therapeutic benefits of melatonin are numerous. Melatonin is a hormone that does much more than regulates the sleep cycle. It has been used as a therapy for Alzheimer's disease, stroke, traumatic brain injury, COVID-19, heart health, hypertension, memory loss, and even preoperative anxiety. It also has been effective therapy for the following disorders.

● **Breast Cancer.** Melatonin demonstrates both cytostatic (inhibits cell growth and division) and cytotoxic (toxic to the cell) activity in breast cancer cells. To be specific, the anti-cancer actions of the circadian melatonin signal in human breast cancer cell lines and xenografts heavily involve MT1 receptor-mediated mechanisms. In estrogen receptor positive human breast cancer, melatonin suppresses ER alpha mRNA expression and ER alpha transactivation activity through the MT1 receptor. Also, melatonin controls the transactivation of other members of the nuclear receptor superfamily, estrogen-metabolizing enzymes, and the expression of core clock and clock-related genes.

Furthermore, melatonin also suppresses tumor aerobic metabolism (the Warburg effect previously described) and, subsequently, cell-signaling pathways critical to cell proliferation, cell survival, metastasis, as well as drug resistance. Furthermore, melatonin has anti-invasive/anti-metastatic actions that involve many pathways, including inhibition of p38 MAPK and repression of epithelial-mesenchymal transition). Studies have demonstrated that melatonin promotes genomic stability by inhibiting the expression of LINE-1 retrotransposons which are a type of genetic component that copy and paste themselves into different genomic locations (transposon) by converting RNA back into DNA through the reverse transcription process using an RNA transposition intermediate.

Finally, research has indicated that light at night induced disruption of the circadian nocturnal melatonin signal promotes the growth, metabolism, and signaling of human breast cancer and drives breast tumors to endocrine and chemotherapeutic resistance. These data provide the strongest understanding and support of the mechanisms that underlie the concept of elevated breast cancer risk in night-shift workers and anyone else that is exposed to light at night.

Many studies have shown, moreover, that melatonin is an effective therapy for breast cancer as an adjunct to traditional care. It has also been shown to be effective in the prevention and reduction of some of the side effects of chemotherapy and radiation including mouth ulcers, dry mouth, weight loss, nerve pain, weakness, and thrombocytopenia (low platelet count). Moreover, melatonin has been used as a therapy for other cancer forms such as brain, lung, prostate, head and neck, and gastrointestinal cancers.

- **Gastrointestinal Diseases.** The enterochromaffin cells of the gastrointestinal tract secrete 400 times as much melatonin as the pineal gland. Consequently, it is not surprising that numerous studies have found that melatonin plays an important role in GI functioning. As previously mentioned, melatonin is a powerful antioxidant that resists oxidative stress due to its capacity to directly scavenge reactive species, increase the activities of antioxidant enzymes, and stimulate the innate immune response through its direct and indirect actions. In the gastrointestinal tract, the activities of melatonin are mediated by melatonin receptors, serotonin, and cholecystokinin B receptors, as well as through receptor-independent processes.

- **Immune Builder.** Melatonin has been shown to be a major regulator of the immune system. Consequently, disease states affecting a wide range of organ systems have been reported as benefiting from melatonin administration.

- **Insulin Regulation and Obesity.** Melatonin is necessary for the proper synthesis, secretion, and action of insulin. In addition, melatonin acts by regulating GLUT4 expression through its G-protein-coupled membrane receptors, the phosphorylation of the insulin receptor, and its intracellular substrates that mobilize the insulin-signaling pathway. GLUT4 is the insulin-regulated glucose transporter found primarily in adipose tissues (fat tissue) and striated muscle (skeletal and cardiac). Furthermore, melatonin is responsible for the establishment of adequate energy balance by regulating energy flow and expenditure through the activation of brown adipose tissue and participating in the browning process of white adipose tissue. Likewise, melatonin is a powerful chronobiotic, meaning that it helps regulate the body's internal clock.

- **Longevity.** Lab trials have shown that melatonin replacement increases SIRT1, which is a longevity protein. SIRT1 is also activated by caloric restriction.

- **Sleep Hygiene.** Melatonin has long been known to be beneficial for sleep. Melatonin has been shown to synchronize the circadian rhythms and improve the onset, duration, and quality of sleep. The good news is that exogenous melatonin supplementation is well tolerated and has no obvious short- or long-term adverse effects when used in small doses to improve sleep hygiene.

Consequently, the reduction in melatonin production that may occur with aging, shift work, or illuminating environments during the night commonly induces insulin resistance, glucose intolerance, sleep disturbance, and metabolic circadian changes that commonly lead to weight gain. A study using laboratory animals showed that melatonin supplementation daily at middle age decreased abdominal fat and lowered plasma insulin to youthful levels. A low melatonin level is a frequently overlooked cause for an individual's inability to lose weight effectively.

POSSIBLE SIDE EFFECTS AND CONTRAINDICATIONS OF MELATONIN

Melatonin is an immune stimulator. Therefore, it should be used with caution in individuals that are pregnant or breast feeding, patients that have an autoimmune disease, leukemia, or lymphoma, people who suffer from mental illness, and anyone taking steroids.

SIGNS AND SYMPTOMS OF EXCESS MELATONIN

☐ Abdominal pain

☐ Daytime sleepiness/fatigue

☐ Depression

☐ Headaches

☐ Hypotension (low blood pressure)

☐ Increase in cortisol, which can increase fat storage

☐ Intense dreaming/nightmares

☐ Suppression of serotonin, which increases carbohydrate cravings

☐ Transient dizziness

CAUSES OF EXCESS MELATONIN

The most common reason that people have elevated levels of melatonin is that they take doses that are too large, or they take melatonin and do not need it. Likewise, an individual may also have high levels of melatonin if they eat too many foods that contain melatonin. Some medications such as desipramine, fluvoxamine, Thorazine, and tranylcypromine may raise melatonin levels, as can St. John's wort supplementation. Ingesting the herb *Vitex agnus-castus* (chaste tree) can also lead to elevated melatonin levels. If melatonin levels are high, serotonin levels tend to decline. Therefore, it is important to test your melatonin levels, by salivary testing, if you are taking more than one mg of melatonin at night.

MELATONIN DOSING SCHEDULES

Generally, women are more sensitive to melatonin than men if melatonin is being suggested for insomnia. Some women may need only a very low dose, and hence the melatonin may need to be compounded. In addition, medical studies have also suggested that patients may need less melatonin for insomnia as they age. As previously mentioned, large doses of melatonin are used to treat breast cancer and other cancers. For breast cancer therapies: 12 to 20 mg, 30 to 60 minutes before bedtime. One suggested protocol for breast cancer patients is the following:

● Stage I breast cancer: 3 mg one hour before bedtime

● Stage II breast cancer: 6 mg one hour before bedtime

● Stage III breast cancer: 12 mg one hour before bedtime

● Stage IV breast cancer: 20 mg one hour before bedtime

SUMMARY

Melatonin is a wonderful hormone that has so many functions in the body aside from regulating sleep. As you have seen, it has been shown to be an effective treatment for many disease processes along with a beneficial way to build the immune system. In addition, it has been shown to be an effective therapy to prevent breast cancer as well as treat all stages of breast cancer in conjunction with traditional therapies.

THYROID HORMONES

Your thyroid gland is more important than you might think. You probably are aware that you have a thyroid gland, but chances are that you may not know the major role it plays in the complex workings of your body. The thyroid gland regulates almost everything that occurs in your system. It is, in fact, the conductor of the wonderful symphony that occurs daily in your body. There are several different thyroid hormones that your body synthesizes. They are:

- Diiodothyronine (T2)
- Triiodothyronine (T3)
- Thyroxine (T4)
- Reverse triiodothyronine (rT3)

T2. T2 increases the metabolic rate of your muscles and fat tissues. T2 stimulates cellular/mitochondrial respiration and outside the cell affects the carriers, ion-exchanges, and enzymes. It may also affect the transcription of genes.

T3. This hormone is four to five times more active than T4. T3 is about 20 percent of the thyroid hormone production by the body. It affects most of the physiological processes in the body, except for the spleen and testes. This hormone increases basal metabolic rate, oxygen, and energy consumption by the body. It is very important for weight loss and to break down cholesterol. It even affects the production of serotonin in the brain, which is your happy neurotransmitter. T3 furthermore increases the rate of protein synthesis and affects glucose metabolism. The T3 hormone is available in two forms: bound T3 which is attached to protein and free T3 which does not attach to anything. When you have your T3 measured, your healthcare provider should measure the free form.

T4. T4 is 80 percent of the thyroid gland's production. Most of T4 is converted into T3 in your liver or kidneys, so some authors suggest that T4 is really a prohormone (a steroid). T4 is responsible for increasing cardiac output, increasing basal metabolic rate, and increasing heart rate and ventilation. It also potentiates the effect of catecholamines (a type of hormone that strongly affects blood pressure) and thickens the endometrium of the uterus in women. T4 can also be converted into rT3 which is an inactive (stored) form. The T4 hormone is also available in two forms: bound T4 which is attached to protein and free T4 which is not bound. When you have your T4 measured, your healthcare provider should measure the free form.

rT3. Reverse triiodothyronine (rT3) is created by the body from T4. It is an anti-thyroid metabolite that blocks T3 from working in your body.

FUNCTIONS OF THE THYROID GLAND AND THYROID HORMONES

The thyroid gland is a key gland producing hormones that play a major part in the human body's everyday workings. These hormones:

- Affect tissue repair and development
- Aid in the function of the mitochondria (energy makers of your cells)
- Assist in the digestion process by regulating GI tone and motility
- Control hormone secretion and therefore regulate fertility, ovulation, and menstruation
- Control oxygen utilization by regulating resting respiratory rate and minute ventilation
- Modulate blood flow
- Regulate carbohydrate, protein, and lipid metabolism
- Modulate muscle and nerve action
- Modulate sexual function
- Regulate energy and heat production through blood flow, sweating, and ventilation
- Regulate growth and repair
- Regulate vitamin usage, for example, by promoting folate (B_9) and cobalamin (B_{12}) absorption through the GI tract
- Regulate cardiac output, stroke volume, contractility, and resting heart rate
- Regulate basal metabolic rate (BMR)
- Promote oxygen delivery to the tissues by simulating erythropoietin and hemoglobin production

- Stimulates the nervous system resulting In Increased wakefulness, alertness, and responsiveness to external stimuli.

- Stimulates the peripheral nervous system resulting in increased peripheral reflexes

- Regulates kidney clearance of many substances including medications can be increased due to an increase in renal blood flow and glomerular filtration rate

- Increase development of type II muscle fibers

The thyroid gland can become overactive (hyperthyroidism) or underactive (hypothyroidism) which affects your well-being resulting in several issues including increasing your risk of developing breast cancer. Below are signs and symptoms of low thyroid function and also symptoms of an overactive thyroid.

SIGNS AND SYMPTOMS OF HYPOTHYROIDISM

Early diagnosis of hypothyroidism isn't always easy. Most people with an underactive thyroid aren't aware that they have this condition. They may suffer a number of symptoms without recognizing that the symptoms are thyroid-related or that there may be no symptoms early on in the disease process. Often, the healthcare provider may minimize or misdiagnose the symptoms. Clinical manifestations of hypothyroidism range from life threatening to no signs or symptoms. The signs and symptoms of hypothyroidism normally progress slowly, over months or years, and quite often they may be confused with other disorders. The following are signs and symptoms of hypothyroidism:

☐ Acne

☐ Agitation/irritability

☐ Allergies

☐ Anemia (normocytic)

☐ Anxiety/panic attacks

☐ Bladder and kidney infections

☐ Blepharospasm (eye twitching)

☐ Bradycardia (slow heart rate)

☐ Carpal tunnel syndrome

☐ Cholesterol levels that are high (hypercholesterolemia)

☐ Cognitive decline

☐ Cold hands and feet

☐ Cold intolerance

☐ Congestive heart failure

☐ Constipation

- [ ] Coronary heart disease/acute myocardial infarction (heart attack)
- [ ] Course facial features
- [ ] Decreased cardiac output
- [ ] Decreased sexual interest
- [ ] Delayed deep tendon reflexes
- [ ] Deposition of mucin (glycoprotein) in connective tissues
- [ ] Depression
- [ ] Dizziness/vertigo
- [ ] Downturned mouth
- [ ] Drooping eyelids
- [ ] Dry skin
- [ ] Dull facial expression
- [ ] Ear canal that is dry, scaly, and may itch
- [ ] Ear wax build-up in the ear canal (cerumen)
- [ ] Easy bruising
- [ ] Eating disorders
- [ ] Elbows that are rough and bumpy (keratosis)
- [ ] Endometriosis
- [ ] Erectile dysfunction
- [ ] "Fat pads" above the clavicles
- [ ] Fatigue
- [ ] Fibrocystic breast disease
- [ ] Fluid retention
- [ ] Gallstones
- [ ] Goiter
- [ ] Hair loss in the front and back of the head
- [ ] Hair loss in varying amounts from legs, axilla, and arms
- [ ] Hair that is sparse, coarse, and dry
- [ ] Headaches, including migraine headaches
- [ ] High cortisol levels
- [ ] High C-reactive protein (CRP)
- [ ] Hoarse, husky voice
- [ ] High homocysteine levels (hyperhomocysteinemia)
- [ ] High insulin level (hyperinsulinemia)
- [ ] High prolactin level
- [ ] High triglycerides
- [ ] Hypertension (high blood pressure)
- [ ] Hypoglycemia (low blood sugar)
- [ ] Impaired kidney function
- [ ] Inability to concentrate
- [ ] Increased appetite
- [ ] Increased LDL (bad cholesterol)
- [ ] Increased risk of developing asthma
- [ ] Increased risk of developing bipolar disorder
- [ ] Increased risk of developing schizoid or affective psychoses

☐ Increased creatinine kinase (indicative of muscle damage)

☐ Infertility

☐ Insomnia

☐ Joint stiffness

☐ Lethargy (lack of energy and enthusiasm)

☐ Loss of eyelashes or eyelashes that are not as thick

☐ Loss of one-third of the eyebrows

☐ Low amplitude theta and delta brain waves

☐ Low blood pressure

☐ Low body temperature

☐ Macroglossia (enlarged tongue)

☐ Menstrual cycle pain

☐ Menstrual irregularities including abnormally heavy bleeding (menorrhagia)

☐ Mild elevation of liver enzymes

☐ Miscarriage

☐ Morning stiffness

☐ Muscle and joint pain

☐ Muscle cramps

☐ Muscle weakness

☐ Muscular pain (myalgia)

☐ Nails that are brittle, easily broken, ridged, striated, thickened nails

☐ Nocturia (need to get up and urinate in the middle of the night)

☐ Nutritional imbalances

☐ Osteoporosis (bone loss)

☐ Paresthesia (abnormal sensation of feeling burning, tingling, and itching)

☐ Pericardial effusion (buildup of too much fluid in the double-layered saclike structure around the heart (pericardium)

☐ Periorbital edema (fluid build-up around the eyes)

☐ Pleural effusion (accumulation of excess fluid in the pleural space which is the potential space that surrounds each lung)

☐ Poor circulation

☐ Poor night vision

☐ Premenstrual syndrome (PMS)

☐ Proteinuria (abnormal quantities of protein in the urine)

☐ Puffy face

☐ Reduced heart rate

☐ Rough, dry skin

☐ Shortness of breath

☐ Sleep apnea

☐ Slow movements

☐ Slow speech

☐ Swollen eyelids

☐ Swollen legs, feet, hands, and abdomen

☐ Tendency to develop allergies

☐ Tinnitus (ringing in the ears)

☐ Vitamin B$_{12}$ deficiency

☐ Voice changes

☐ Weight gain

☐ Yellowish skin discoloration due to the inability to convert beta carotene into vitamin A

SIGNS AND SYMPTOMS OF HYPERTHYROIDISM

The following are the most common signs and symptoms of hyperthyroidism. The progression of these individual symptoms, however, may also differ from one individual to another. It is also important to keep in mind that many of these signs and symptoms can be caused by other underlying problems.

Early Symptoms

☐ Anxiety, nervousness, and irritability

☐ Brittle fingernails

☐ Breast enlargement in men (rare)

☐ Bulging eyes (exophthalmia)

☐ Constipation

☐ Diarrhea and/or an increase in bowel movements

☐ Difficulty in managing diabetes

☐ Elevated heart rate (tachycardia) and/or chest pain

☐ Erectile dysfunction or reduced sexual urges

☐ Eyelid retraction, puffy eyelids, reddening around the eyes, pressure on the eyes, and irritation of the eyes as well as double vision (Graves' thyroid eye disease) Goiter (enlargement of the thyroid gland) Heart palpitations (sensation heart is pounding)

☐ Heat or cold intolerance

☐ Muscle weakness

☐ Personality or psychological changes Perspiring profusely (diaphoresis) Separation of nail from the nail bed (onycholysis) Shortness of breath

☐ Skin changes

☐ Slight trembling of the hands or fingers

☐ Weight change (weight loss or gain)

Late Symptoms

☐ Decreased ability to hear

☐ Hoarseness, lumpy thickening and reddening of the skin, usually on the shins or tops of the feet (Graves' dermopathy)

☐ Menstrual disorders

☐ Puffy face, hands, and feet

☐ Slow speech

☐ Thinning eyebrow hair

If you have any of the above symptoms, see your healthcare provider to have your thyroid hormones tested. It is important that your doctor measures all the following studies and not just one or two of them.

STANDARD BLOOD TESTS

Normally, every blood test you take includes a group of tests that look at your body's hormones. It typically analyzes your thyroid hormones including TSH, free T3, free T4, reverse T3, and the thyroid antibodies; antithyroglobulin, anti-microsomal, antithyroperoxidase and thyroid-stimulating hormone receptor. The results are printed on your blood test lab report.

Thyroid-stimulating hormone (TSH). It measures the amount of TSH in the blood. TSH is produced by the pituitary gland in the brain. It is responsible for regulating the amount of hormones released by the thyroid gland.

• Free T3 and Free T4. These levels measure the free hormone in the blood which is not bound and able to enter and affect the body tissues.

• Reverse T3. This level is the body's ability to store free T3 for a "rainy day." Stored Reverse T3 means you cannot use it and even though your level of free T3 could be within the normal range, you still may experience hypo-thyroid symptoms.

• Thyroid antibodies.

SUMMARY

Hopefully, you have come to understand the critical role that the thyroid gland and its hormones play to sustain the many systems that keep you alive and functioning normally but also in its relationship to breast cancer. If you or a loved one suffers from some of the symptoms described above, and you have not been able to isolate their cause, I hope you consider acting as an advocate and asking your healthcare provider to determine if these symptoms are thyroid related. Make sure that your doctor does all of the tests described in this section of the chapter.

CONCLUSION

Many of us hear the word "hormone" and think of estrogen for women and testosterone for men. We know they are important for our sexuality, but that's about it. Few of us understand what they do, or for that matter, understand how important all of our body's hormones are. The fact is that our hormones allow our body's systems to function. They provide pathways and communication to tell every part of our body to carry on life. When just one of our hormones overproduces or underproduces, the balance of our hormones is thrown off, creating a multitude of health problems.

In this chapter, we have looked at all the major hormones—where they come from, what they do, and what happens if they are thrown out of balance. Many of us experience several common health issues such as headaches, anxiety, insomnia, indigestion, dry skin, and consider them problems of daily life. What we don't realize is that the majority of them are caused by one or two of our hormones missing the mark. When these struggles become chronic, we go to a healthcare provider to have them checked out through salivary testing and blood testing. However, in some cases, it is important to recognize some of these troubles before they become chronic, so that they don't develop into something more serious such as breast cancer. By recognizing the signs and symptoms of these problems, and knowing what you can do to alleviate them, you also have the ability to increase your odds of not getting breast cancer.

7

Controllable Health Disorder Risk Factors

There are certain illnesses and health conditions that have been shown to increase a woman's risk of developing breast cancer—and as we will see, many of these risks may seem trivial. We simply accept them as part of our normal lives. The doctor tells you your cholesterol is somewhat high, or you make a promise to yourself to lose those extra pounds, but you just let it go for one more year. But what we don't realize is that they all have more of an impact on the way our body behaves than we realize. The more you do to control your health, the more likely you are to decrease your risk of developing breast cancer.

GASTROINTESTINAL (GI) TRACT HEALTH

Your GI tract is part of your overall digestive system. It is made up of the mouth, the esophagus (food pipe), the stomach, and the large and small intestines. The health of your GI tract has a great deal to do with whether you develop breast cancer and whether you can *beat* breast cancer. Seventy percent of your immune system is in your GI tract. (See page 218 on immunity.) In fact, the human microbiome in the gut plays an integral role in physiology with most microbes considered benign or beneficial. However, some microbes are known to be detrimental to human health, including organisms linked to cancers and other diseases characterized by inflammation.

As you read this part of the book, it is important to understand two terms that sometimes are used interchangeably; however, they do not really mean the same thing. Human *microbiota* is the term used to describe all the microorganisms (bacteria, eukaryotes, archaea, and viruses) within the human body; in other words, the community of microorganisms themselves. The *microbiome* is defined as the complete catalog of these microbes and their genes; in other words, the collective genomes of the micro-organisms in a particular environment.

Dysbiosis occurs in your GI tract when there is a state of microbial imbalance. When this happens, harmful bacteria compete with benign bacteria, which can lead to maladies (including cancer). Furthermore, pre-existing imbalance in the gut has been reported as a host-intrinsic regulator of tissue inflammation and tumor cell dissemination in breast cancer. Moreover, a study investigating differences in gut microbiome composition among postmenopausal women showed a less diverse fecal microbiome and a significantly altered composition in newly diagnosed breast cancer individuals compared with healthy controls. These findings suggest an unrecognized link between dysbiosis and breast cancer, which has potential diagnostic and therapeutic implications.

In addition, data indicates that an alteration of the function of the microbiota by antibiotics may have negative impacts on breast cancer patient outcomes. This is important since antibiotics are regularly prescribed to breast cancer patients undergoing mastectomy or breast reconstruction. Therefore, the metabolic impact of disruption to the microbiome should be considered alongside the significant immunological effects.

The gut bacterial microbiome includes an *estrobolome*. The estrobolome is a collection of bacteria in the gut, capable of breaking down and regulating the body's circulating estrogen. It has a key influence on a woman's lifetime exposure to major estrogens. The bacterial composition of the estrobolome, in turn, is likely affected by age and ethnicity, as well as lifetime environmental influences including diet, alcohol, and antibiotic use—all of which affect bacterial populations. Some of these factors have also been independently linked to breast cancer risk.

Estrogens are primarily produced in the ovaries, adrenal glands, and adipose tissue and circulate in the bloodstream in free or protein-bound form. Estrogens are responsible for many different chemical reactions in the body. These chemical reactions carry on many important functions in the body. (See Chapter 6, "Controllable Hormonal Risk Factors," page 104.) This process is referred to as *metabolism*. They first undergo metabolism in the liver, where estrogens and their metabolites (the different chemicals produced during these reactions) are put together.

This mixture of metabolites, called *conjugated estrogens*, are eliminated from the body by metabolic conversion to water-soluble molecules, which are excreted in urine or in bile into the feces with the help of an enzyme called *beta-glucuronidase* (part of the estrobolome). This then leads to the reabsorption of estrogen back into the circulation that affects other tissues, including the breast (where it stimulates the growth of cells). Consequently, the estrobolome affects both the elimination and circulation of estrogen—and also the reabsorption back into the body.

Recent research suggests that the microbiota (set of living organisms that inhabit the intestine) of women with breast cancer differs from that of healthy women, indicating that certain bacteria may be associated with cancer development and with different responses to therapy. Furthermore, microbiomes are different in the four forms of breast cancer: *endocrine receptor (ER) positive*, *triple positive, Her2 positive*, and *triple negative breast cancers*. Studies have shown that there are distinct patterns for the triple negative and triple positive samples, while the ER positive and Her2 positive samples shared similar microbial signatures. These signatures provide a new line of investigation to gain further insights into prognosis, treatment strategies, and clinical outcomes, as well as better understanding of the role of microorganisms in the development and progression of breast cancer.

Moreover, the microbiota-mediated regulation of innate and adaptive immune responses to tumors (see Chapter 9, "Looking Forward," page 283, for more on the immune system), and the consequences on cancer progression and whether tumors subsequently become resistant or susceptible to different cancer therapies are related to the ratio of healthy to non-healthy bacteria in the GI tract. Consequently, let's explore how your GI tract works and what therapies are available to promote optimal health of your gut.

THE GASTROINTESTINAL TRACT

Your gastrointestinal tract (GI tract) is literally 70 percent of your immune system. In the GI tract can be found the largest blood supply in the body, using one-third of the total blood flow from the heart. The gut flora contains 400 different microbial species. Consequently, the gut has a massive amount of influence on your metabolism. It is really a hidden organ! It has greater metabolic activity than the liver, with ten times the number of cells and 100 times the genomic material. The cells of the intestinal tract are shed and replaced every three to six days. Therefore, they are very sensitive to nutrition and lifestyle choices.

Function of the GI Tract

Therefore, if your gut is not healthy—then *you* are not healthy. Dr. Jill Carnahan is one of the gurus in the world concerning GI health. She states the following: "You are what you eat, and then absorb, and then what you do or do not detoxify." What does the GI tract do in the body? The following are the major functions of the GI tract:

- **Digestion.** This is the process whereby our food is broken down into smaller portions that are more easily absorbed by the intestines.

- **Absorption.** This is the process whereby the digested food is taken up by the intestine and delivered to the body for utilization as energy, nutrition, and other cellular functions.

- **Detoxification.** This is the complex process (involving the liver and GI tract) whereby toxins are metabolized for elimination from the body. Toxins include such things as: the medication(s) we take that must be metabolized; to pesticides, preservatives, dyes, and flavor-enhancers we ingest knowingly in our food; as well as the over 4 million chemicals present in our environment that are not intended for use in our bodies. In addition, 25 percent of the estrogen that the body makes—as well as 25 percent that is used as a medication—is detoxified through the GI tract. Consequently, if the gut is not healthy it increases your risk of developing breast cancer.

- **Elimination.** After digestion has occurred, and the metabolic phase of detoxification is complete, the GI tract must then eliminate the digestive and metabolic wastes of these processes. Some refer to this as *excretion*. Transit time in the intestine from mouth to rectum should be 24 to 30 hours. In the US, it is about 48 hours. One-fourth of the estrogen produced by the body is eliminated after it is metabolized (broken down) in the GI tract.

- **Exclusion.** This refers to the barrier function performed by the GI tract, as it appropriately excludes substances from entering the body.

GI Microbiome and the GI Barrier

How do you have a healthy gut? From a traditional medicine viewpoint, you have a healthy GI tract when you have met these five major criteria: *effective digestion and absorption of food, absence of GI illness, normal and stable intestinal microbiota, effective immune status,* and *status of well-being*. There is now ample evidence that two functional entities are also key to achieving and maintaining gut health. These entities are the GI microbiome and the GI barrier, which is not just a mechanical barrier assessed by permeability measurements.

Multiple functions of the GI microbiome have been described. The GI microbiome prevents colonization by potentially pathogenic microorganisms, provides energy for the gut wall from undigested food, and regulates the mucosal immune system. Most importantly, the GI microbiota contributes to the maintenance of an intact GI barrier, which is closely related to infectious, inflammatory, and allergic diseases.

The *gastrointestinal mucosa*—membrane rich in mucus—forms a barrier between the body and potential hostile microorganisms and toxins. In addition, the GI barrier allows the stomach to safely store the gastric acid that is necessary for digestion.

INTESTINAL DYSFUNCTION

Almost half of the adults in the US experience intestinal illness at some time in their lives. Even emotional trauma can negatively impact your digestion. Dr. D. L. Berkson wrote the number one best-selling book of all time on GI health, *Healthy Digestion the Natural Way*. The following are signs of poor digestion and then optimal digestion—it may surprise you that to have perfect digestion, you need to have two normal bowel movements a day.

Signs of Poor Digestion

☐ Chronic indigestion after eating

☐ Chronically coated tongue

☐ Depressed without a reason

☐ Feeling better if you do *not* eat

☐ Feeling stress without a cause

☐ Foul-smelling stools

☐ Frequent burping, flatulence, and/or bloated stomach

☐ Frequently cold for no reason

☐ Increase in pulse of 20 to 25 beats within 15 minutes after eating

☐ Less than one bowel movement a day

☐ Needing to loosen your belt after eating (even though you did not overeat)

☐ Poor sleeping habits/waking up tired

☐ Undigested food in stools

Signs of Optimal Digestion

☐ Do not have frequent mood swings, shakiness, anxiety, or depression without a reason

☐ Feeling better after exercising

☐ Feeling good after eating and several hours later

☐ Good energy level throughout the day

☐ No extreme food cravings

☐ No undigested food in stools

☐ Sleeping well (and waking up rested)

☐ Stools do not smell

☐ Two bowel movements a day

☐ Warm extremities

The GI tract needs basic nutrients: B vitamins, such as B_1, B_6; folic acid; and also vitamins A, C, D, and E. The gut also needs minerals, such as zinc, selenium, manganese, molybdenum, magnesium, and the amino acid arginine. Therefore, starting with a good multivitamin that is pharmaceutical-grade is a great place to start your journey to optimal GI health.

■ DYSBIOSIS (IMBALANCE IN THE GUT)

Dysbiosis is an inflammatory disease of the GI tract caused by an imbalance of intestinal bacteria. The consequences of dysbiosis are great, including loss of good bacteria and loss of the production of some important vitamins. In addition, the gastrointestinal tract is one of the body's five organs of detoxification. Consequently, if you have dysbiosis, your body does not detoxify well. Furthermore, dysbiosis can cause you to lose protection from chemical toxins and antibiotics (along with having a subsequent overgrowth of harmful bacteria). Recent studies indicate that dysbiosis increases your risk of developing breast cancer. (See Chapter 8, "Strengthening Your Immune System," page 233, for further discussion on this subject.)

Symptoms of Dysbiosis

Many symptoms can occur due to dysbiosis, including ones that are related to both inside and outside the GI tract, extraintestinal symptoms, which Dr. Berkson brilliantly discusses in her book.

Common symptoms include:

- ☐ Abdominal distention and bloating
- ☐ Abdominal pain
- ☐ Altered bowel function (constipation and/or diarrhea)
- ☐ Belching
- ☐ Bloating
- ☐ Cramping
- ☐ Cramps and spasms
- ☐ Flatulence
- ☐ Halitosis
- ☐ Heartburn
- ☐ Hypersecretion of colonic
- ☐ Mucus
- ☐ Nausea

Extraintestinal symptoms linked to dysbiosis include:

- ☐ Anxiety
- ☐ Brain fog
- ☐ Cognitive and memory deficit
- ☐ Depression
- ☐ Fatigue
- ☐ Fever of unknown origin

☐ Frequent urination

☐ Joint pain

☐ Inflammation in the vein

☐ Itching

☐ Malaise

☐ Muscle pain

☐ Palpitations

☐ Seizures

☐ Skin rashes

☐ Vasculitis

Causes of Dysbiosis

The causes of dysbiosis are numerous. Consequently, it is a common problem. It is often due to one, or a combination, of the following:

- Alcohol abuse
- Carbohydrate malabsorption
- Consumption of infected foods
- Corticosteroid use
- Diminished bile
- Excessive stress
- Food allergies and sensitivities
- Free radical production
- Gastrointestinal surgeries
- Hypoxia/exposure to extreme altitude
- Immune deficiencies
- Improper fasting or dieting
- Low levels of hydrochloric acid in the stomach
- Nutritional deficiencies
- Pancreatic insufficiency
- Repeated use of antibiotics
- Travel
- Use of non-steroidal anti-inflammatory drugs (NSAIDs)

- Damage the mucosal lining
- Damage the mitochondria (turn energy from food into energy the cell can use)
- Breakdown intercellular integrity
- Recirculated waste products from the liver
- Yeast infections
- Ethanol and acetaldehyde (one of the breakdown products of ethanol) disrupt the tight junctions in the cells lining the intestines which increases membrane permeability.
- Artificial sweeteners cause glucose intolerance by altering the gut microbiota and induce dysbiosis
- Lectins are protein fragments of foods that are not completely digested that bind with specific sugars on the surface cells throughout the body. They stick to the lining of the GI tract, which causes inflammation and can destroy cell membranes.

Lectins flatten the intestinal villi and consequently decrease the absorption of nutrients.

- Activate neutrophils caused by the escape of bacteria and large molecules of undigested food through the compromised intestinal barrier

- Viruses like rotaviruses have proteins on their outer surfaces that can open the cellular spaces between the tight junctions of the GI mucous cells

■ SMALL INTESTINAL BOWEL OVERGROWTH (SIBO)

The GI tract holds a balance of trillions of cells, including bacteria, viruses, and fungi. It just has to be the right kind of bacteria and the right number of bacteria. An imbalance of this complex intestinal microbiome, both qualitative and quantitative, may have serious health consequences for the body, including *small intestinal bowel overgrowth*, commonly called SIBO. This is a specific kind of dysbiosis.

SIBO is defined as an increase in the number and/or alteration in the type of bacteria in the upper gastrointestinal tract, where it does not belong. This overgrowth of bacteria usually only occurs in the colon, which is part of the large intestine. The body has mechanisms for preventing bacterial overgrowth: gastric acid secretion, intestinal motility, intact ileocecal valve, immunoglobulins within intestinal secretion, and bacteriostatic properties of pancreatic and biliary secretion. In some people, more than one cause may be involved in the development of SIBO.

Symptoms

Symptoms related to SIBO are:

- ☐ Abdominal pain
- ☐ Diarrhea
- ☐ Malnutrition
- ☐ Bloating
- ☐ Malabsorption
- ☐ Weight loss

The diagnosis is made by an upper GI aspirate or three-hour lactulose breath test for hydrogen/methane.

Causes

SIBO is commonly the cause of a (motility) movement problem in the small intestine. If something impairs movement, such as one or more of the following, the small intestine cannot eliminate the bacteria:

- Achlorhydria (low stomach acid)

- Excessive use of antibiotics

- Gastrointestinal conditions (irritable bowel syndrome, inflammatory bowel disease, and celiac disease)

- History of bowel surgeries or anatomical abnormalities (small intestinal obstruction, diverticula, fistulae, surgical blind loop, previous ileocecal resections)

- Immunodeficiency syndromes

- Impaired valve separating the small and large intestines (ileocecal valve)

- Long-term use of proton pump inhibitors (PPIs)

- Motility disorders (scleroderma, autonomic neuropathy in diabetes mellitus, post-radiation enteropathy, small intestinal pseudo-obstruction)

- Pancreatic exocrine insufficiency

- Poor gallbladder function

- Poor nutrient status (deficiencies of choline, taurine, magnesium, and others)

Therapies

Small intestinal bowel overgrowth therapies are designed to correct the balance of bacteria in the small intestines. Doctors begin treating SIBO by examining the cause of the underlying disease. Nutritional therapies and even antibiotics are also commonly required.

Medications

Therapies for SIBO may include medications such as:

- *Rifaximin* is an antibiotic that fights a bacterial infection only in the intestine. If you are a methane producer, your doctor may add metronidazole or neomycin. Low dose erythromycin may be useful.

- *Prokinetic* medications are also commonly prescribed, which enhance GI motility by increasing the frequency or strength of contractions.

- *Low dose naltrexone* is a novel anti-inflammatory agent with promising immunomodulatory effects. (See later in this book under "Inflammation" for more information.)

Herbal Therapies

The following therapies, for one to two months, are also commonly employed:

- Berberine: 500 mg., three times a day
- Oregano: 200 mg., three times a day
- Garlic extract: 450 mg., twice a day
- Peppermint herb (*Menthae piperitae folium*)

Probiotics

Initially, probiotics may be contraindicated because SIBO often involves an overgrowth of D-lactate-producing bacteria. Therefore, probiotics may be added a couple of weeks later. It is important not to eat two hours before bed-time, and to have four to five hours between meals.

Diet

A SIBO diet should consist of foods high in fiber and low in sugar.

▓ LEAKY GUT SYNDROME

If you have dysbiosis, including SIBO, this commonly leads to *leaky gut syndrome*. Leaky gut syndrome occurs when there is damage to the lining of the bowel, which results in increased permeability. Intestinal permeability is a term describing the control of material passing from inside the gastrointestinal tract through the cells lining the gut wall and then into the remainder of the body.

The intestine normally exhibits some permeability, which allows nutrients to pass through the gut, while also maintaining a barrier function to keep potentially harmful substances from leaving the intestine and moving to the remainder of the body. Increased permeability allows toxins to re-enter the bloodstream and also, if you are taking medication, to possibly get the medication a second time.

Symptoms and Signs

Symptoms and signs of a leaky gut may include:

- ☐ Abdominal pain
- ☐ Anxiety
- ☐ Aches and pain in joints
- ☐ Asthma
- ☐ Aggressive behavior
- ☐ Bedwetting

☐ Bladder infections   ☐ Food sensitivities

☐ Bloating   ☐ Gas

☐ Chronic fatigue   ☐ Indigestion

☐ Chronic joint pain   ☐ Inflammatory skin conditions

☐ Confusion   ☐ Learning disorders

☐ Constipation   ☐ Mood swings

☐ Cramps   ☐ Muscle pains

☐ Diarrhea   ☐ Nervousness

☐ Exercise intolerance   ☐ PMS

☐ Fatigue   ☐ Recurring infections

☐ Fever of unknown cause   ☐ Shortness of breath

☐ Foggy thinking   ☐ Skin rash

Causes of Increased Intestinal Permeability

There is no single cause for leaky gut syndrome, but there are several possible reasons for its development. Some of the underlying causes of leaky gut include:

- Aging process
- Celiac disease
- Chronic alcoholism
- Diarrhea
- Food allergies
- Inflammatory bowel disease
- NSAIDs drugs
- Nutritional depletions
- Protozoal infections
- Small intestinal bacterial overgrowth (SIBO)
- Strenuous exercise
- Stress
- Toxic exposure

Conditions Associated With Leaky Gut Syndrome

Multiple diseases may emerge or be amplified due to a leaky gut, and they may extend beyond the gastrointestinal tract (including breast cancer). Many people have a GI tract that is unhealthy. The good news is that the 5R program for gut restoration can help almost all individuals have a healthy gut, which produces a healthy immune system.

THE 5R PROGRAM FOR GUT RESTORATION

The 5R program for gut restoration was developed by the Institute for Functional Medicine. It is a complete and comprehensive approach that not only improves symptoms, but it helps heal with long-lasting results. The aim of the program is: to address dietary changes; to normalize digestion and absorption; to balance gastrointestinal bacteria; to create a balanced system of detoxification; and to promote healing of the gut.

The following five key points are involved in the 5 R program: Remove, Replace, Repopulate, Repair, and Rebalance. A comprehensive 5 R program takes roughly about three to six months to complete. It is essential that you are amenable to implement the challenging dietary changes of the program; as without the dietary portion, you cannot attain the maximum therapeutic benefit.

It is therefore *crucial* to start the gut restoration program by eating a healthy diet. One study has shown that your diet has the most powerful influence on gut microbial communities, more than anything else that can be done if you are basically healthy to begin with.

1. REMOVE

The first step in helping to achieve optimal GI health is to *remove* anything that has a negative impact on the gut. Finding a trigger may not be initially obvious and, therefore, may take some time. Triggers may include the following:

- **Food allergies.** Food allergies or sensitivities are a common item. At least 60 percent of Americans have food allergies. Food allergy testing that examines both allergies that are IgG- and IgE-related may be beneficial to have performed.

- **Pathogens.** Pathogens are organisms that are not desirable, such as yeast, parasites, or pathogenic bacteria. You may need to take medication, such as antibiotics, anti-parasitic agents, or antifungal drugs. Herbal therapies may also be beneficial but commonly require six months of therapy to be effective.

- **Stress.** Both physical and mental stress can negatively impact GI health. Changes that may occur include food cravings and appetite, alterations in gut function, and modifications to intestinal permeability.

- **Medications and supplements.** Medications and supplements can cause gut dysfunction. The most common medications are non-steroidal anti-inflammatory drugs (NSAIDs).

- **Environment.** Environmental stressors that are toxins in the environment can contribute to the toxic load carried by the body and thus can have a negative impact on the GI tract.

- **Inflammation.** Systemic inflammation increases intestinal permeability. (A further discussion on this subject is available elsewhere in this book.)

2. REPLACE

Once the offending agents are removed, the next step is to replace digestive secretions that are low or lacking in your body. You may be deficient in several elements that are fundamental to digestion, such as stomach acid, bile, and digestive enzymes. You also may be lacking in certain nutrients. The following are digestive factors that may be important—and may need replacement.

■ DIGESTIVE ENZYMES' DEFICIENCY

Digestion decreases with age because digestive enzyme production declines, which slows down or inhibits your ability to process nutrients. This may also occur if you do not chew your food well. Studies have shown that you should chew each bite of food 20 times for adequate digestion and production of digestive enzymes. Digestive enzymes have many functions in the body. They enhance digestive health, reduce autoimmunity, decrease post-surgery recovery time by decreasing the need for pain relievers, and reduce swelling. In fact, digestive enzymes are used in Europe (due to their anti-inflammatory effect) to treat arthritis.

SIGNS AND SYMPTOMS OF PANCREATIC ENZYME DEFICIENCY

An increase in meat and vegetable fibers in your stool suggests impaired digestion due to insufficient pancreatic enzymes or low HCL levels. There are many signs and symptoms of pancreatic enzyme deficiency:

☐ Fat-soluble vitamin deficiencies

☐ Food intolerances

☐ Gastroesophageal reflux

☐ Hypochlorhydria (low stomach acid)

☐ Loose or watery stools

☐ No improvement in health when eating a good diet and taking supplements

☐ Postprandial bloating, pain, or nausea one half-hour to several hours *after* eating (low stomach acid produces pain immediately after eating)

☐ Undigested food in stool

Evaluating Pancreatic Insufficiency

Measuring *pancreatic elastase* (PE) levels is a reliable method for the evaluation of pancreatic insufficiency. PE is a proteolytic enzyme secreted exclusively by the human pancreas. It reflects overall enzyme production (amylase, lipase, and protease) and is not affected by gut transit time, not enzymatically degraded, and not affected by digestive enzyme supplementation.

Enzyme Depletion

Lifestyle choices and aging can be a factor in the body's ability to produce the needed enzymes, as well as certain conditions.

- Arterial obstruction
- Bovine growth hormone used in red meat
- Celiac disease
- Cooking foods at high temperatures
- Fluoridation of water
- Heavy metals
- Hybridization and genetic engineering of plants
- Inflammatory disorders
- Ischemic disease
- Lactose intolerance
- Large intake of unsaturated and hydrogenated fats
- Malabsorption
- Maldigestion
- Mercury amalgam dental fillings
- Microwaving
- Pancreatic insufficiency
- Pasteurization
- Pesticides
- Radiation and electromagnetic fields
- Rheumatoid arthritis
- Root canals and hidden dental infections
- *Steatorrhea* (excess fat in feces)

Digestive Enzymes' Replacement

Take two to three digestive enzymes just before or at the very beginning of a meal.

Bitters: Bitters trigger the release of digestive enzymes in the mouth. They also increase the release of HCL in the stomach and enhance the production of bile. In addition, bitters increase the production of saliva and gastric juices, which accelerate the natural emptying of the stomach and cause the pancreas to release digestive enzymes. Bitter herbs have been shown to treat the following conditions: sluggish digestion, flatulence, bloating, dyspepsia, and bowel distention. There are commercially formulated bitters. In addition, a salad with dandelion leaves, escarole, endive, and other bitter salad greens, which can be combined with romaine lettuce, is an excellent way to get bitters into your diet.

Enzymatic Therapy Replacement. Enzymatic therapy replacement is a medical treatment in which the enzyme level is increased. It has been shown to be effective for many conditions.

Side Effects and Contraindications

Do not take digestive enzymes if you have ulcers, or any kind of active inflammatory bowel condition, without first consulting your healthcare provider. If the digestive enzyme contains papain and you are on the blood-thinner medication Coumadin, then do not take it. Some digestive enzymes contain papain from papaya to assist in protein digestion. Do not use any digestive enzymes that contain papain if you are allergic to papaya.

Speak to your doctor or pharmacist to learn if any drugs you are taking might make it unwise to use digestive enzymes. Avoid enzymes with bromelain if you are allergic to pineapple, latex, wheat, celery, carrot, fennel, cypress pollen, or grass pollen. Furthermore, high doses of digestive enzymes can negatively impact uric acid levels. Although relatively rare, the side effects of digestive enzymes can also include the following: constipation, cough, diarrhea, gas, heartburn, nausea, upset stomach, and/or even a sore throat.

▓ GASTRIC ACID (BETAINE HCL)

Gastric acid, a source of hydrochloric acid, has two major functions. It sterilizes the food and also increases the digestive enzymes if taken with food to improve digestion and to help heal leaky gut syndrome. However, if the digestive enzymes are taken on an empty stomach they will have an anti-inflammatory action. It also increases the denaturing proteins—breaking of many of the weak hydrogen bonds within a protein molecule—which prepares the protein for breakdown by gastric and pancreatic enzymes.

Cause

Low levels of hydrochloric acid (*hypochlorhydria*) in the stomach are caused by: widespread use of antacids (which are the third most common OTC medication); prescription drugs that block stomach acid production; the aging process; and genetic causes. Low stomach acid is also more common in individuals who are vegetarian, and in people who fast regularly. In fact, if you have any debilitating chronic condition, it increases your risk of low stomach acid.

SIGNS AND SYMPTOMS OF LOW STOMACH ACID

The possible consequences of low stomach acid are significant, including major mineral deficiencies (calcium, magnesium, zinc, iron, chromium, manganese, copper, and molybdenum). Furthermore, B_{12} deficiency is a possible side effect of low stomach acid. In addition, you may have even more signs and symptoms if you have low stomach acid, such as:

- ☐ Acne
- ☐ Bloating or belching immediately after meals
- ☐ Chronic intestinal infections
- ☐ Dilated blood vessels in the cheeks and nose
- ☐ Multiple food allergies
- ☐ Muscle cramps and spasms
- ☐ Rosacea
- ☐ Undigested food in your stools
- ☐ Upper digestive tract gassiness

Diseases/Conditions Linked to Low Levels

Maintaining low levels of stomach acid can bring about a range of distressing side effects, and leave the body exposed to the development of several disorders.

Natural Treatments

Therapies for low stomach acid are contingent on the underlying cause. However, there are some approaches you can try at home to improve stomach acid levels. Below are natural ways to increase hydrochloric acid in the stomach:

- • Apple cider vinegar and lemon
- • Betaine HCL (do not use it if you have a peptic ulcer)
- • Bitter herbs
- • Chew food thoroughly
- • Digestive enzymes
- • Enteric-coated peppermint oil

- Garlic
- Ginger
- Glutamine
- Grapefruit seed extract
- Lemons
- Limes

- Multivitamin
- Oregano oil
- Papaya
- Pineapple
- Probiotics
- Vitamin B complex

Work with your healthcare provider to try and avoid use of antacids, PPIs, and H2 receptor antagonists unless you have Barrett's esophagus. If you have Barrett's esophagus, then PPIs should be taken for the remainder of your life. If you and your doctor decide to stop your PPI, you may need to wean off of it due to a possible rebound effect if you have been taking it long-term. If you have an H. Pylori infection, see your doctor or other healthcare providers for treatment.

Protocol for HCL Acid Supplementation

You may need to take HCL acid. Do not take it if you have an active ulcer or have Barrett's esophagus or are actively bleeding anywhere. See a Personalized Medicine or functional medicine specialist for more information.

Bile salts. They are very important in helping to digest fats, fat-soluble vitamins, and essential oils as well as carry waste products from the liver. Bile salts are alkaline and help to maintain adequate bowel flora.

SIGNS AND SYMPTOMS OF LOW BILE SALTS

Low bile salts lead to poor absorption of iron and calcium. The following are signs and symptoms of low bile salts:

☐ Bloating, gas, abdominal discomfort—especially after fatty meals

☐ Chronic constipation

☐ Dull right-sided fullness several hours after eating

☐ Fat soluble vitamin deficiency

☐ Heartburn

☐ Stools that are consistently pale brown, yellowish, or grayish

☐ Vague and intermittent abdominal pains

When you take bile salts, only take them for two months. If symptoms return, then go back on them for another two months and then discontinue them. Excessive replacement can lead to greenish-tinged diarrhea with an unpleasant odor. Bile salts come from animal sources so you can have allergic reactions to them.

High-fiber diet. A diet high in fiber can promote an increase in bacterial richness in the gut, thereby preventing conditions and diseases, such as obesity and metabolic syndrome. Likewise, adding in fiber in several different forms supports bowel transit time and motility which aids in eliminating toxins.

3. REPOPULATE

Repopulation is to restore the balance of good bacteria in your gut which is absolutely crucial to your overall health and having optimal immune function. This phase of the program involves using probiotic foods, fiber-rich foods, and commonly a supplement to help beneficial bacteria flourish.

PROBIOTICS

Begin by repopulating the gut with probiotics, which are good bacteria. They improve the intestinal microbial balance. In addition, reintroduction of good GI *microflora* leaves less space for pathogenic organisms to populate. Specifically, research has found strong associations between strains of *Bifidobacteria* and *Lactobacillus* as well as *Saccharomyces boulardii* and improvements in intestinal cell barrier function and intestinal permeability.

If you have a severely compromised immune system, you should not use live probiotics since the organisms may cross the gut lining and be absorbed. Instead, use the non-live forms of probiotics. Probiotics play a protective role against the colonization of intestinal pathogenic microbes and increase mucosal integrity by stimulating epithelial cells, which are cells that form a barrier between the inside and outside of your body, protecting against viruses. The following are some of the main functions of probiotics for the body.

Functions of Probiotics

Probiotics play a role in restoring your digestive system with good bacteria that will neutralize the harmful microbes. They are believed to:

- Activate regulatory T cells that release IL-10
- Act like natural antibiotics

- Downregulation gut inflammation
- Help digest fats
- Help maintain a beneficial intestinal lining which protects against food allergies
- Help to generate cytokines (proteins that regulate immunity)
- Help with detoxification
- Increase the intestinal and systemic immune response
- Interact with the intestinal epithelial cells (IECs) or immune cells associated with the lamina propria (connective tissue that forms part of the mucous membrane), through Toll-like receptors, and induces the production of different cytokines or chemokines
- Maintain the optimal pH of the intestine
- Make B vitamins
- Make short-chain fatty acids
- Modulate intestinal microbiota by maintaining the balance and suppressing the growth of potential pathogenic bacteria in the gut
- Produce digestive enzymes
- Produce lignins (necessary in the formation of cell walls) to protect against cancer
- Protect against parasites
- Reinforce the intestinal barrier by an increase in mucins (major component of mucus), tight junction proteins, goblet (cells that synthesize and secrete mucus), and paneth cells (cells containing proteins that regulate intestinal flora)

Probiotic Rich Foods and Drinks

The following foods and liquids serve as probiotics:

- Buttermilk
- Essene bread (Ezekiel bread)
- Fermented sausages
- Fermented vegetables
- Ginger
- Kimchee
- Kombucha
- Miso
- Natto
- Olives
- Raw pickles

- Raw vinegars
- Raw whey

- Sauerkraut
- Sourdough

- Tempeh
- Yogurt/kefir

Commonly, as previously discussed, probiotics also need to be taken as a supplement. Supplements should be pharmaceutical-grade and contain several different strains of *Lactobacillus* sp, *Streptococcus* sp, and *Bifidobacterium* sp. Some also contain *S. boulardii*. The probiotics should contain between 20 billion and 100 billion organisms.

PREBIOTICS

After one month on probiotics, you can then begin to take prebiotics (which are agents that support the growth and integrity of the probiotics). In other words, prebiotics are food for good bacteria since they help the growth of beneficial bacteria. They have been reported to improve the expression of tight junction proteins (helps cells form a barrier that stops molecules from getting through), including occludin and zonulin, thereby decreasing intestinal permeability.

Functions of Prebiotics

Prebiotics triggers the growth of health microbes in the gut by:

- Causing a significant change of gut microbiota composition, especially an increase of fecal concentrations of *Bifidobacterium*
- Having a positive effect on energy balance
- Helping with satiety regulation
- Improving general well-being and reduces the incidence of allergic symptoms such as atopic eczema
- Improving stool quality (pH, SCFA, frequency, and consistency)
- Improving the expression of tight junction proteins
- Increasing calcium absorption
- Lowering morning cortisol if it is elevated
- Modulating biomarkers and activities of the immune system
- Reducing the incidence of tumors and cancers
- Reducing the risk of gastroenteritis and infections

Prebiotic Rich Foods

Prebiotic-enriched diets also have been shown to lower inflammatory mediators and decrease oxidative stress as well as increase the production of beneficial short-chain fatty acids such as butyrate. The following are prebiotic rich foods:

- Asparagus
- Burdock root
- Chicory
- Cottage cheese
- Eggplant

- Garlic
- Green tea
- Honey
- Jerusalem artichokes
- Kefir

- Leeks
- Legumes
- Onions
- Peas
- Yogurt

Furthermore, prebiotics improve glucose sensitivity and help to eliminate body fat as well as lower blood pressure and help to eliminate toxins. They also improve liver function and reduce serum cholesterol. Like probiotics, prebiotics are available commercially in the form of fructo-oligosaccharides (FOS), guar, lactulose, and inulin. Prebiotics are also available in many foods that contain inulin, such as garlic, onions, legumes, chicory, soybeans, asparagus, garlic, and leeks.

You may need to take probiotics and prebiotics for the remainder of your life. The best way to permanently change the gut microbiota in your body is to eat a healthy diet.

4. REPAIR

The gut lining can be severely damaged during times when the body is inflamed, under stress, and exposed to long-term allergens. This increases the intestinal permeability of the gut which allows antigenic macromolecules to cross the gut epithelium (gut tissue) leading to chronic systemic inflammation, which then decreases the gut bacteria leading to leaky gut syndrome. Repair of the GI tract lining is needed to ensure proper absorption of nutrients as well as medications.

THERAPIES

Repairing the GI lining requires several therapies. Begin by eating a diet rich in amino acids, vitamins, and minerals. The following therapies have also been shown to be beneficial:

- Anti-inflammatory agents such as fish oil, which can reverse intestinal dysbiosis, and curcumin, which improves barrier function.

- Chamomile (*Matricaria chamomilla*) has anti-inflammatory action that is due to azulene and bisabolene, which are two chemicals in chamomile. Its name means "mother of the gut." In Germany it is an OTC licensed drug for treatment of GI spasms and inflammatory diseases of the GI tract.

- Chinese skullcap (*Scutellaria baicalensis*) contains baicalin and wogonin, which have anti-inflammatory action by blocking the arachidonic acid cascade and it helps heal the gastric mucosa.

- Citrus flavanones can regulate the microbiota composition, as indicated in recent evidence, and activity by inhibiting pathogenic bacteria and selectively stimulating the growth of good bacteria. Citrus flavanones, with hesperidin and naringin as the most abundant representatives, also have various beneficial effects, including anti-oxidative and anti-inflammatory activities. In addition, the consumption of citrus flavanones has been associated with a lower risk of degenerative diseases, such as cardiovascular diseases and cancers.

- Demulcents are herbs or foods that have a protective effect on the mucous membranes of the body. They contain a large amount of mucilaginous materials that have a direct effect on the lining of the intestines to soothe them. Likewise, demulcents also reduce the sensitivity of the digestive system to gastric acids, relax spasms, decrease leaky gut, inflammation, and ulceration. The following are examples of demulcents: cabbage juice, Fenugreek (*Trigonella foenum-graecum*), Marshmallow (*Althea officinalis*), Okra (*Hibiscus esculentus*), and Slippery elm bark (*Ulmus fulva*).

- Ginkgo biloba has been shown to protect the integrity of the mucosal lining of the intestines by reducing oxidative damage.

- Goldenseal (*Hydrastis canadensis*) stimulates the immune response and destroys germs since it contains berberine. It also has astringent effects that aid in digestive problems and is used to treat peptic ulcers and colitis. Goldenseal, in addition, promotes the production and secretion of digestive juices and helps to reestablish healthy gut mucosa. Barberry or Oregon grape root, which are berberine-rich substitutes, can also be used.

- Glutamine is an amino acid that stimulates intestinal mucosal growth and protects the gut from mucosal atrophy. It also plays an important role in acid-base balance and has an immunomodulating effect by increasing IL-6 levels and lymphocyte function. However, glutamine is a precursor to glutamate or glutamic acid. Glutamate is one of two excitatory neurotransmitters in the brain that can cause anxiety. Consequently, work with your healthcare provider before taking glutamine. Levels of your amino acids can be measured by blood or urine and then you and your doctor can make an informed decision on the use of glutamine for GI health.

- Licorice root (*Glycyrrhiza glabra*), which contains flavonoids called saponin glycosides, have a protective effect on the gut. It has also been shown to decrease GI bleeding secondary to NSAIDs.

- Meadowsweet (*Filipendula ulmaria*), contains glycosides, tannins, mucilage, and flavonoids, which acts as an anti-inflammatory. In addition, it aids in strengthening the bonds of the connective tissue between cells, which helps protect the intestinal barrier. It is also a free radical scavenger.

- Mucosal secretion, such as phosphatidylcholine, plantain, and polysaccharides, protects the respiratory system with lubrication and plays an important role in the allergic inflammatory response.

- Nutrients that are antioxidants, such as carotenoids, and vitamins A, C, D, E, selenium, and zinc along with n-acetyl cysteine (NAC), decrease oxidative stress, which is one of the main causes of intestinal damage.

- Phosphatidylcholine (PC) is a ubiquitous membrane phospholipid that is essential for cellular differentiation, proliferation, and regeneration and is necessary for the transport of molecules through membranes. It has been shown to improve intestinal barrier function. DOSE: 1,000 mg a day. If you have elevated TMAO levels do not take PC.

- Quercetin is a bioflavonoid that is found in onions and blue-green algae. It is an antioxidant and an anti-inflammatory, and it works by decreasing mast cell (acts as an anticoagulant) and basophil (type of white blood cell) production.

- Whey, immunoglobulins, lactoferrin, and lactoperoxidase support gut-associated lymphoid tissue (GALT) function.

ENERGY BALANCE

The ability to repair is also affected by energy balance. Anything that affects ATPase activity (necessary for cell metabolism and exporting toxins) can also affect absorption. The ATPase activity and absorption of nutrients can be impacted by magnesium deficiency, insulin resistance, hypothyroidism (low thyroid function), catecholamine production (hormones and neurotransmitters by the adrenal glands and other organs), and adrenal insufficiency by altering glucocorticoid (steroid) metabolism.

5. REBALANCE

Rebalance, the fifth "R" in the program, is where your way of life plays a crucial role. It is necessary to address the external stressors in your life that may increase your sympathetic drive in the nervous system and reduce the parasympathetic drive. The sympathetic section generally functions in actions requiring quick responses, fight or flight. The parasympathetic section functions with actions that do not require immediate reaction, associated with relaxation, digestion, and regeneration.

With practices like yoga, meditation, deep breathing, good sleep and other mindfulness-based practices, you can help restore hormone balance that will protect your gut and subsequently, your entire body. It would be pointless to go through the first 4 Rs of the gut restoration program to only go back to old eating habits, lack of exercise, stress, and other things that contributed to the GI dysfunction. The 5th R is just as important as the others for optimal GI health.

SUMMARY

In review, a healthy gut flora supports optimal digestion of food, hormone balance, and immune function. It helps to maintain optimal levels of vitamins and minerals, balances neurotransmitter levels, and reduces inflammation. Lastly, one of the principal regulators of circulating estrogens is the gut microbiome. Consequently, in order for the body to break down estrogen and excrete it from the body, the GI tract must be healthy.

The mechanisms of ensuring gut health are complex and comprise a healthy lifestyle, a balanced diet, normal GI perfusion, and normal GI microbiota along with the remainder of the items discussed in this chapter.

This part of the book has explored gut health and metabolic approaches to gastrointestinal (GI) imbalance. There are many causes of digestion and absorption problems. Some are due to mechanical issues, such as mastication, motility, and permeability. Inability to digest effectively may lead to bloating, gas indigestion, constipation, diarrhea, or abdominal complaints. Likewise, GI complaints are due to multifactorial dysfunctions. Abnormal permeability of the intestinal wall can lead to leaky gut syndrome, yeast overgrowth, development of food allergies, and toxin production. Low gastric acidity can lead to symptoms of bloating, belching, burning, and flatulence immediately after ingesting a meal. A deficiency of gastric enzymes may lead to delayed breakdown of protein and result in symptoms of protein maldigestion. Likewise, pancreatic enzymes are required to break proteins into peptides, and a deficiency of proteolytic enzymes (produced by the pancreas and stomach) is another reason that the digestion of protein by the body may not work optimally.

Therapeutic approaches to the restoration of enzymatic function, to reduce inflammation, and balance the microbiota, are key components that are addressed in this section of the text, along with the chapter on inflammation. You now know how to optimize the health of your gut through the "5 R" program of remove, replace, repopulate, repair, and rebalance.

ORAL HEALTH AND BREAST CANCER

One of the risk factors you may not be expecting is that a contributing factor to breast cancer is your oral health. Periodontal diseases comprise a wide range of inflammatory conditions that affect the supporting structures of the teeth (the gingiva, bone and periodontal ligament), which could lead to tooth loss and contribute to systemic inflammation. Periodontal disease begins and progresses through an imbalance of the oral microbiota living in the mouth. This is the dental plaque, that is, the film of bacteria that builds up on teeth, which can then interact with your immune defenses leading to inflammation and disease. Specifically, the severity of the periodontal disease depends on environmental and host risk factors, both controllable like smoking and those that are unchangeable such as genetic susceptibility.

Studies reveal that periodontal disease contributes to the development of breast cancer. In fact, women who suffer from gum disease are up to three times as likely to develop breast cancer according to a recent study. Periodontal disease may affect the initiation and development of breast cancer involving microorganisms and inflammation which may originate in the infected gums and/or from the bacteria in the mouth that may enter the circulation through the gums which can then affect the tissue of the breast. Consequently, implementing ways to prevent and treat periodontal disease is of great importance. Moreover, periodontal health is affected by radiotherapy, chemotherapy, and endocrine therapy for breast cancer. In particular, the structures of the oral cavity are influenced by estrogen; therefore, anti-estrogen therapies may negatively impact your oral health. Regular visits to your dentist will help prevent periodontal disease and help you maintain optimal oral health.

DENTAL SIDE EFFECTS FROM BREAST CANCER TREATMENTS

Based on the type of treatment used to combat breast cancer, there may be a number of problems that may directly affect your teeth and mouth. The use of certain chemotherapies may stop the salivary glands from producing enough saliva leading to dry mouth which can cause gum disease and cavities. This may also produce breeding gums. Chemotherapies can also suppress the immune system making a patient susceptible to infections in the mouth or bloodstream.

When dental work is necessary and you are being treated for breast cancer, make sure you tell your dentist about the cancer treatment you are undergoing before any work is done on your teeth.

HIGH CHOLESTEROL (HYPERCHOLESTEROLEMIA)

High cholesterol (hypercholesterolemia) is a risk factor for ER-positive breast cancer (cancer cells grow in response to estrogen). Instead of cholesterol, the cholesterol metabolite 27-hydroxycholesterol induces the proliferation of estrogen receptor-positive breast cancer cells and facilitates metastasis. More-over, oxidative modification of lipoproteins and HDL glycation (attachment of a sugar to a protein) activate different inflammation-related pathways. Thereby, enhancing cell proliferation (rapid increase in numbers) and migra-tion spread and inhibiting apoptosis (cell death).

In addition, vitamin D supplementation has been shown to decrease cir-culating 27-hydroxycholesterol (27HC) in breast cancer patients most likely by inhibiting CYP27A1 (protein coding gene). Inhibition of CYP27A1, the enzyme responsible for the rate-limiting step in 27-hydroxycholesterol biosynthesis, significantly reduced metastasis (cancer spread) in several studies.

Cholesterol is a wax-like fatty substance—a lipid—found in the cell mem-branes of all body tissues. About 75 percent of it is synthesized by the body, with the rest being of dietary origin. Despite cholesterol's bad reputation, it is actually necessary for proper body function, and plays a central role in many biochemical processes, including the production of sex hormones. But at the same time, excessively high levels of cholesterol—referred to as hypercholes-terolemia—pose a threat to good health.

There are two major forms of cholesterol:

1. High-density lipoproteins (HDLs) which are often referred to as "good cho-lesterol," carry cholesterol from the blood to the liver for elimination from the body.

2. Low-density lipoproteins (LDLs), or "bad cholesterol," carry cholesterol from the liver to the rest of the body.

Your *total cholesterol* considers both LDL and HDL levels because they are both important for good health. When there are high levels of LDLs in the blood—and especially when this is accompanied by low levels of

HDLs—cholesterol can be deposited on the walls of the arteries, causing atherosclerosis (hardening of the arteries). This condition, in turn, is the underlying cause of strokes, heart attacks, and most cardiovascular disease in general.

CAUSES OF HIGH CHOLESTEROL

The following are some of the causes of total high cholesterol.

- Alcoholism
- Amino acid deficiency
- Biotin deficiency
- Carnitine deficiency
- Deficiency of natural antioxidants, such as vitamin E, selenium, and beta-carotene

- Essential fatty acid deficiency
- Excess dietary starch
- Excess dietary sugar
- Fiber deficiency
- Food allergies

Hypercholesterolemia is also linked to high *triglyceride* levels. This refers to the form that fat takes when it is being stored for energy in your body. Triglycerides, like cholesterol, are vital for human life but unhealthy if they reach too high a level. Your doctor will be able to test your HDL, LDL, and triglyceride levels by taking a simple blood test. (You may need to fast the day of the test. Your doctor will provide you with details.)

Dietary changes are key to lowering both cholesterol and triglycerides. Red meat and other foods high in saturated fats should be eaten sparingly, while heart-healthy fish, vegetables, fruits, grains, and nuts should be included in greater amounts. Soy foods, which decrease LDL cholesterol and triglycerides, should also be featured in your diet. There are also a number of supplements that can decrease your cholesterol levels.

Exercise is vital to achieving and maintaining healthy cholesterol levels. Additionally, certain nutrients such as those listed in the table "Supplements That Decrease Cholesterol Levels" can help lower bad cholesterol, raise good cholesterol, and restore heart health.

SUPPLEMENTS THAT DECREASE CHOLESTEROL LEVELS		
Supplements	Dosage	Considerations
Alpha-lipoic acid	400 to 600 mg once a day	Alpha-lipoic acid can interact with medication taken for diabetes and thyroid problems. Speak to your healthcare provider to see if any of the medications you take make it unwise to use this supplement.

Supplements	Dosage	Considerations
Astragalus*	250 to 500 mg standardized	Do not use after organ transplant or if you have an extract three to four times a day allergy to gum tragacanth. Also do not use for an extended period of time. Speak to your healthcare provider to see if any of the medications you take make it unwise to use astragalus.
B-complex vitamins	50 mg twice a day	I suggest taking a multivitamin along with your B-complex vitamins.
Carnitine*	500 to 3,000 mg once a day	Have your healthcare provider measure your TMAO levels before starting long-term supplementation with carnitine.
Coenzyme Q_{10}*	100 to 400 mg once a day	If you are on blood-thinning medications, speak to your healthcare provider before using CoQ_{10}. Since some medications can cause a deficiency of this nutrient, speak to your healthcare provider to determine if you might need a larger dose.
Cysteine	1,000 mg once a day as n-acetylcysteine, or NAC	When taking NAC supplements, also take extra vitamin C, copper, and zinc.
Lysine	1,000 to 3,000 mg once a day	Do not take if you have diabetes or are allergic to eggs, milk, or wheat. Do not take for more than six months because it can cause an imbalance of arginine unless arginine is also supplemented.
Milk thistle	100 to 200 mg twice a day	Do not take if you are allergic to ragweed, chrysanthemums, marigolds, chamomile, or daisies. This supplement reduces the efficiency of certain blood pressure medication and other drugs. Speak to your healthcare provider or pharmacist before taking.
Olive leaf extract*	500 mg to 750 mg a day containing 20 mg of oleuropein per capsule	Olive leaf extracts can interact with many prescription medications, and may increase the effects of blood thinners. Consult your healthcare provider before using olive leaf extract if you are taking any medication. Don't use if you are pregnant or breastfeeding.
Phosphatidylcholine (PC)	2,000 to 10,000 mg once a day	Use with caution if you have malabsorption problems, as this could exacerbate them.
Probiotics	20 billion units once a day	If taking an antibiotic, take the probiotics at least two hours before or two hours after using the antibiotics. Do not take them at the same time.
Selenium	200 mcg once a day	Do not exceed 200 mcg a day without consulting your healthcare provider.

Supplements	Dosage	Considerations
Taurine	1,000 to 3,000 mg	Take between meals. Discontinue use if you suddenly have feelings of chest or throat tightness or if you break out in hives. Do not take with aspirin. Have your healthcare provider measure levels before starting taurine therapy.
Vitamin B_9 (folic acid)	500 mcg twice a day	High doses can deplete your body of other B vitamins, so take a B-complex vitamin twice a day.
Vitamin B_{12} (cobalamin)	500 to 1,000 mcg twice a day	High doses can deplete your body of other vitamins in the B complex, so take a B-complex vitamin twice a day.
Vitamin C	500 to 2,500 mg twice a day	Do not take high doses if you are prone to kidney stones or gout. High doses can also cause diarrhea.
Vitamin D_3	Have your blood levels measured by your healthcare provider, who will determine proper dosage.	
Vitamin E*	400 IU once a day	Take mixed tocopherols, the more active type of vitamin E. Consult your healthcare provider first if you are taking a blood thinner.
Vitamin K*	45 mg a day of K_2	This dose has been shown to help prevent the development of liver carcinoma in women with cirrhosis due to chronic hepatitis. If you are on a blood thinner, do not take vitamin K except under the direction of your doctor.

*CAUTION: Be aware that these supplements can have a blood-thinning action.

SUMMARY

As previously discussed, breast cancer is the most prevalent cancer and primary cause of cancer-related mortality in women. The identification of risk factors can improve prevention of cancer, and hypercholesterolemia represents a potentially controllable breast cancer risk factor. This section explored the progress to date in research on the potential role of the main cholesterol transporters, low-density and high-density lipoproteins (LDL and HDL), on breast cancer development. The cholesterol substance produced during metabolism, metabolite 27-hydroxycholesterol (27HC), has been shown to possess estrogenic activities related to estrogen and to promote breast tumor growth in animal and human trials in both pre- and postmenopausal women through several mechanisms.

Although some studies have failed to find associations between lipoproteins and breast cancer, some large clinical studies have demonstrated a direct association between LDL cholesterol levels and breast cancer risk and an inverse association between HDL cholesterol and breast cancer risk.

Fortunately, there are many ways to lower cholesterol which is becoming increasingly important, not just to prevent heart disease, but also to prevent breast cancer and to help prevent a reoccurrence.

INFECTION

For many years, breast cancer has been suggested in the medical literature to be possibly tied to infection. Viral, bacterial, and fungal infections have all been suggested. Studies reveal that infection by microbial species as a risk factor is responsible for initiating 2.2 million new cancer cases a year. Many of these are breast cancer. Chronic inflammation is believed to be the common pathway through which infections increase the risk of breast cancer development. The mechanism of chronic inflammation leading to cancer development and progression is not specific to bacteria. Other microorganisms like viruses and fungi can also promote an inflammatory pathway leading to cancer metastasis.

VIRAL INFECTIONS

There are several viruses that have been linked to breast cancer development over the years. Since the discovery, decades ago, of the oncogenic mouse mammary tumor virus (MMTV), there has been significant interest in the potential role of infectious agents as a cause of sporadic human breast cancer. To address this, many studies have examined the presence of viruses (for example, papillomaviruses, herpes viruses, and retroviruses), endogenous retroviruses and more recently, microbes, as a means of implicating them in the cause of human breast cancer. Unfortunately, the trials have generated conflicting reports of the role of infection in breast cancer.

Recently, however, there has been a resurgence of interest in the possibility that a significant proportion of human breast cancers may be caused by viral infections. Several viruses have been proposed.

- A human retroviral analogue of mouse mammary tumor virus (MMTV) which occurs in up to 37 percent of individuals with breast cancer.

- Mouse mammary tumor virus has also been suspected. MMTV DNA sequences have been found in 36 percent of human breast tumor samples and 24 percent of non-cancerous breast tissue. It is related to BRCA1 breast cancer.

- Oncogenic human papillomaviruses (HPVs) have been found in breast cancers in 30 studies conducted in 17 countries and four continents. HPV prevalence in breast cancer in published reports ranges from 0 percent to 86 percent.

- Epstein-Barr virus (EBV), also called human herpesvirus 4 (HHV-4) is one of eight members of the herpes family. Detection rates of EBV in breast cancer range from 0 percent to 68 percent.

- Bovine leukemia virus (BLV) is a retrovirus. In one study of 114 U.S. breast cancers, 59 percent were positive for BLV when compared with 29 percent of 104 normal breast controls. The source of BLV infection may be cows' milk.

- Severe coronavirus diseases 2019 (COVID-19) cause a hyperactivation of immune cells, resulting in lung inflammation. Recent studies showed that COVID-19 induces the production of factors previously implicated in the reawakening of dormant breast cancer cells. Further studies will be required to confirm the link between COVID-19 and cancer reoccurrence.

FUNGAL INFECTIONS

Fungi were found to promote the growth of tumors in different parts of the body including the breast. In particular, the fungus Malassezia yeast has been linked to reduced survival rates in breast cancer.

BACTERIAL INFECTIONS

It is now estimated that around 16 percent of all cancers are related to microbial infections and toxicities. Breast cancer is one of these cancers.

Various bacterial species, their virulence factors, and their role in cell transformations leading to cancer (particularly gastric, oral, colon, and breast cancer) are now being researched. Bacterial imbalance penetrates into host cells, causes inflammation, and results in the development of tumors. Bacterial-mediated host cell transformations cause chronic inflammation, immune receptor hyperactivation/absconding immune recognition, and genomic instability. Bacterial infections reduce the number of E-cadherin (a cell adhesion molecule found in normal breast tissue), which plays a crucial role in breast cancer metastases, with worse prognosis, and shorter overall survival.

It is important to understand that it is proposed that microbial infection not only can boost the cancer risk but conversely can also serve as a treatment. Consequently, although uncovering and comprehending the association between bacteria and cancer is highly challenging, it also may serve as a successful cancer therapy in the future.

The emergence of bacteriotherapy, which is the treatment of disease using bacteria, combined with conventional therapies is now leading to new and effective ways of overcoming cancer treatment challenges. The combination of bacteriotherapy and conventional therapy has shown significant and sustained therapeutic potential. Conventional chemo/radiotherapy is associated with a possible relapse of tumors and adverse side effects due to their lack of specificity and systemic toxicity. Thus, bacteria therapy combined with chemo/radiotherapy may be a new approach to overcome these drawbacks.

SUMMARY

Recent trials have shown that infection has a role in the development of breast cancer. Fungi, bacteria, parasites, and viruses have all been linked to the development of this form of cancer. In addition to understanding the role of bacterial infections in cancer development, the application of bacteria for cancer therapy is an inviting area of study. Moreover, the breast itself has its own microbiomes.

INFLAMMATION

Short-term inflammation protects the host cells by fighting the foreign organisms, but long-term inflammation can lead to cancer development. Several studies showed that chronic inflammation acts as a driving force in cancer development, intensifying malignant transformation, tumor growth, invasion, and metastasis. About 25 percent of human cancer is associated with chronic inflammation. Inflammation shows greater replicative potential and self-determination of growth factors. Furthermore, the ability to stop growth is also absent in inflammation conditions. Chronic inflammation contributes to the malignant transformation—process that a cell goes through to become a rapidly dividing tumor-producing cell of several malignancies and is an important component of breast cancer.

The findings from David N. Danforth and others at the National Institute of Health indicate that in healthy normal breast tissue there is systemic evidence to suggest inflammatory changes are present and associated with an increase in breast cancer risk. Interestingly, the microbiome, genomic abnormalities, and cellular changes are present in healthy normal breast tissue, with the potential to initiate inflammatory changes. Chronic inflammation over time can cause damage to cell DNA and affect the way cells grow and division which could promote the growth of tumors and lead to breast cancer.

These findings suggest that chronic inflammation may play a role in influencing the initiation, development, and conduct of breast cancer, although several chronic inflammatory processes in breast tissue may occur later in the course of the disease. Breast cancer is an inflammatory disease process. This is evidenced by an increase in inflammatory markers that can occur in breast cancer such as c-reactive protein (CRP). A meta-analysis demonstrated that elevated plasma CRP levels were associated with an increased risk for breast cancer. Moreover, among premenopausal women, high TNF-alpha (another inflammatory marker) was associated with a significantly increased risk in developing breast cancer.

DECREASE INFLAMMATION

Breast cancer is an inflammatory disease process. Lowering the level of inflammation in your body decreases your risk of developing breast cancer. There are many articles that extensively demonstrate the direct relationship between chronic inflammation and cancer. In fact, inflammation is often associated with the development and progression of cancer. The cells responsible for cancer-associated inflammation are genetically stable and thus are not subjected to rapid emergence of drug resistance.

Inflammation can occur from outside the body caused by infection, toxins, cigarette smoking, and excessive alcohol intake. All of these, as you have seen, increase your risk of cancer and stimulate the spread of the disease. Conversely, inflammation can originate inside the body from mutations and can contribute to the progression of breast cancer. Moreover, both forms of inflammation can suppress the immune system and provide an environment for tumor development.

Several pro-inflammatory gene products have been identified that mediate a critical role in suppression of apoptosis, proliferation, angiogenesis, invasion, and metastasis. The expression of these pro-inflammatory gene products is mostly regulated by the transcription factor NF-kappa B, which is active in most tumors and is induced by carcinogens (such as cigarette smoke), tumor promoters, carcinogenic viral proteins, chemotherapy, and gamma-irradiation. Consequently, several studies have identified nuclear factor-kappa B as a key modulator in driving inflammation in cancers. Consequently, these observations suggest that anti-inflammatory agents that suppress NF-kappa B or NF-kappa B-regulated products should have potential in both the prevention and treatment of cancer since chronic inflammation caused by biological, chemical, and physical factors have been found to increase the risk of developing breast cancer.

Moreover, obesity is an inflammatory process and increases the risk of many cancer types including breast cancer. Obesity is also associated with poor outcomes. Furthermore, inflammatory processes induce oxidative stress and reduce cellular antioxidant capacity due to overproduced free radicals which react with cell membrane fatty acids and proteins impairing their function long-term. In addition, free radicals can lead to mutation and DNA damage that can be a predisposing factor for cancer and age-related disorders.

Likewise, microbes are critical regulators of the host immune system and, ultimately, of inflammation. Consequently, microbes have the potential power to influence tumor progression as well, through a wide variety of routes, including chronic activation of inflammation, alteration of tumor microenvironment, and damage to DNA. Part of the inflammation that occurs is due to an imbalance between the types of organisms present in a person's natural microflora in the GI tract. Therefore, having a healthy gut, as discussed in a previous section, decreases your risk of developing breast cancer by decreasing inflammation and helping to build your immune system. Now, let's examine the inflammatory process further.

WHAT CAUSES INFLAMMATION IN THE BODY?

Before the body sets up an inflammatory response, the immune system must recognize a threat to the body from one or more of the following categories that are discussed at length in Dr. Nancy Appleton's book entitled: *Stopping Inflammation: Relieving the Cause of Degenerative Diseases.*

- Microbial infections: viruses, bacteria, parasites, fungi infections can set up an inflammatory response by secreting various white blood cells

- Surgery: of any type including oral surgery

- Physical agents: tissue damage can occur due to trauma, ultraviolet or other forms of radiation, burns, or frostbite

- Vaccinations: all cause an inflammatory response

- Chemicals: from household cleaners, products at work, pesticides, products during traveling

- Disease processes: most diseases after the age of 45 and many diseases when you are younger

- Smoking and other tobacco use sets up an inflammatory response

- AGEs: advanced glycation end products are a source of inflammation from the diet and eating processed foods

- Free radical production that causes oxidative stress, creating inflammation

- Obesity: the more overweight you are the more inflamed you are

- Chronic fatigue: stress on the body which produces inflammation

- Allergies: to foods, spices, and environmental vehicles, such as trees, animal dander, pollen

In addition, other causes of inflammation have also been discussed in the medical literature such as dairy products, mitochondrial damage, abnormal sleeping patterns, an unhealthy diet, even some medications and physical inactivity.

WHAT HAPPENS TO THE BODY IN AN INFLAMMATORY REACTION?

The primary goal of the inflammatory response is to detect and eliminate factors that interfere with homeostasis. A typical inflammatory response consists of four components: inflammatory inducers; detecting sensors; downstream mediators; and the target tissues that are affected.

The type and the degree of inflammatory response activated is dependent on the nature of the inflammatory trigger (bacterial, viral, or parasitic) and its persistence. The body produces substances to try and decrease the inflammation and attempt to heal itself.

A healthy person produces circulating immune complexes. They are made up of foreign invaders or antigen and white blood cells called antibodies. The following are some of the inflammatory mediators produced by the body: chemokines, cytokines, eosinophils, free radical production, insulin, interleukins, leukotrienes, mast cells, prostaglandins, and serotonin.

Cytokines play a large role in breast cancer related to inflammation. Several cytokines regulate the inflammatory tumor microenvironment. Interleukin (IL)-1, IL-6, IL-11, and transforming growth factor-β (TGF-β) stimulate cancer cell proliferation and invasion and cytokine receptor activation and intracellular signaling by NF-κB accelerate tumor progression. TGF-β is the most extensively studied cytokine in breast cancer. TGF-β belongs to the TGF-β superfamily and is a major regulator of many processes, including proliferation, differentiation, migration, immunity, and apoptosis. TGF-β has two actions in tumor progression. As a tumor suppressor, it has anti-proliferative effects in the early stages of tumorigenesis, but tumor cells in later stages evade this effect and progress in response to this cytokine.

Physical Changes

The classic signs of inflammation are heat, redness, swelling, pain, and loss of function. These are manifestations of the physiological changes that occur during the inflammatory process.

Chemical Mediators

Chemical mediators of the inflammatory process include a variety of substances originating in the plasma and the cells of uninjured tissue, and possibly from the damaged tissue. A hormonal response also occurs where hormones such as cortisol are produced, which have an anti-inflammatory effect. Some other hormones have a pro-inflammatory effect. Thus, the endocrine system has a regulatory effect on the process of inflammation so that it can be balanced and beneficial in the body's attempts to recover from injury or infection.

■ LEAKY GUT SYNDROME AND INFLAMMATION

Leaky gut syndrome results from continuous damage to the gastrointestinal tract (GI) from inflammatory processes due to infection, to antibiotic use, to food allergies. If your GI tract is not healthy, commonly there is inflammation being displayed as part of this reaction. When you suffer from a leaky gut, bacteria and toxins enter the bloodstream and can cause inflammation and may bring about a reaction from the immune system. *See* the above section on GI health for a more extensive discussion.

■ ADVANCED GLYCATION END PRODUCTS (AGEs)

There are also other forms of inflammation that are important to further examine. Advanced glycation end products (AGEs), found in protein-rich and sugar-rich foods, can attack any part of the body and mimic a low-grade infection. Advanced glycation end products are proteins or lipids that become glycated as a result of exposure to sugars. They are a biomarker implicated in aging and the development, or worsening, of many diseases.

Conditions Caused by AGEs

AGEs accumulate naturally as you age, and high levels have been connected to the development of many diseases. The following are conditions that can be caused by AGEs. Once AGE products are formed, they are not reversible. As glycation begins, free radicals form in glycated products at five times the rate of non-glycated proteins. Free radicals produce inflammation and oxidative stress.

▓ FREE RADICALS

Immune cells produce free radicals while fighting off antigens that are invading the body. A free radical is a molecule that contains an unpaired electron which is in search of another electron to stabilize the molecule. Free radicals include reactive oxygen and nitrogen species, which are key players in the initiation and progression of tumor cells and enhance their metastatic potential. In fact, they are now considered a hallmark of cancer. However, both reactive oxygen and nitrogen species may contribute to improving the outcomes of radiotherapy in cancer patients.

Sources of Free Radical Production

Although free radicals are produced naturally in the body, factors contributing to your environment and lifestyle influence their production. There are general factors such as aging and chronic stress. Dietary factors also play a role such as a large sugar intake. Chemical factors can cause inflammation from chemical pollutants to even flying in an airplane. Inflammation that is unregulated creates free radical production.

The overproduction of free radicals is known to cause several chronic diseases including cancer. The initiation of cancer in humans caused by reactive oxygen species (ROS) is further supported by the presence of oxidative DNA modifications in cancer tissues. Oxidative DNA damage leading to the development of breast cancer has also been reported. For instance, in inflammatory breast cancer, an increase in DNA base damage and 8-oxo-dG adducts lead to malignant cancer progression.

ROS also induces modifications of redox-sensitive amino acid residues in regulatory proteins including cysteine oxidation. Such modifications can control the regulatory effects of proteins and enzymes. The regulatory proteins such as kinases (MAPK and PI3K/Akt), transcription factors (Nrf2, AP-1, NF-κB, STAT3, and p53) are susceptible to altered physiological function by ROS. These modifications in the regulatory proteins of non-cancerous cells are not able to control cellular balance and as a consequence lead to initiation of carcinogenesis. Stimulation of these signaling pathways by ROS is also found to be involved in growth, migration, and invasion of breast and many other cancer cells. However, it is a two-edged sword, increased production of free radicals by chemotherapeutic drugs is also associated with the death of cancer cells, indicating the dual nature of free radical production.

▓ DISEASES RELATED TO INFLAMMATION

Inflammation plays a central role in healing, but chronic inflammation raises the risk of certain diseases.

Tumor Development

Inflammatory responses play decisive roles at different stages of tumor development, including initiation, promotion, malignant conversion, invasion, and metastasis. Inflammation also affects immune surveillance and responses to therapy. Immune cells that infiltrate tumors engage in an extensive and dynamic crosstalk with cancer cells.

Epigenetic disorders—caused by modifications of gene expression in organisms—such as point mutations in cellular tumor suppressor genes, DNA methylation, and post-translational modifications are needed to transform normal cells into cancer cells. These events result in alterations in crucial pathways that when altered trigger an inflammatory response which can lead to the development of cancer.

Many inflammatory signaling pathways are activated in several types of cancer, linking chronic inflammation to the tumorigenesis process. Immune cells that infiltrate tumors engage in extensive crosstalk with cancer cells. A range of inflammation mediators, including cytokines, chemokines, free radicals, prostaglandins, growth and transcription factors, microRNAs, and enzymes as, cyclooxygenase and matrix metalloproteinase, collectively act to create a favorable microenvironment for the development of tumors.

COMMON TESTS FOR INFLAMMATION

There are now several blood tests that your healthcare provider can order that will help determine if your body is inflamed. Such tests should be performed regularly as a preventative action and to monitor your inflammatory standing.

- **CRP blood test.** C-reactive protein levels rise acutely in response to inflammation following IL-6 secretion by macrophages and T cells. Its physiological role is to bind to the surface of dead or dying cells (and some types of bacteria) in order to activate the complement system.

- **Interleukin-6 blood test.** Interleukin-6 (IL-6) is an interleukin that acts as both a pro-inflammatory cytokine and an anti-inflammatory myokine mediated through its inhibitory effects on TNF-alpha and IL-1. This blood test helps to evaluate conditions, such as lupus, rheumatoid arthritis or even infection, which is linked to inflammation.

- **TNF-alpha blood test.** TNF-alpha is a cell signaling protein (cytokine) involved in systemic inflammation and is one of the cytokines that makes up the acute phase reaction. It is produced chiefly by activated macrophages, although it can be produced by many other cell types, such as T helper cells, natural killer cells, neutrophils, mast cells, eosinophils, and neurons.

- **Cytokine profile test.** Cytokines include chemokines, interferons, interleukins, lymphokines, and tumor necrosis factors. Cytokines are produced by a broad range of cells, including immune cells like macrophages, B lymphocytes, T lymphocytes and mast cells, as well as endothelial cells, fibroblasts, and various stromal cells—cells found in bone marrow. They act through cell surface receptors and they modulate the balance between humoral and cell-based immune responses. Cytokines are involved in host immune responses to infection, inflammation, trauma, sepsis, cancer, and reproduction.

- **Interleukin-2 blood test.** Interleukin-2 (IL-2) is an interleukin, a type of cytokine signaling molecule in the immune system. It regulates the activities of white blood cells (leukocytes and lymphocytes) that are responsible for immunity, and it is part of the body's response to microbial infection. The major sources of IL-2 are activated CD4+ T cells and activated CD8+ T cells.

- **Leukotriene test.** Leukotrienes are a family of eicosanoid inflammatory mediators produced in leukocytes by the oxidation of arachidonic acid (AA) and the essential fatty acid eicosapentaenoic acid (EPA). Leukotrienes regulate immune responses and their production is usually accompanied by the manufacturing of histamine and prostaglandins, which also act as inflammatory mediators. Depending on what country you live in, different tests are available to measure leukotrienes in the body.

- **Erythrocyte sedimentation rate (sed rate).** Sed rate is a common blood study that is a non-specific measure of inflammation.

- **Fibrinogen blood test.** Fibrinogen is an acute-phase protein produced by the liver. Its blood levels rise in response to systemic inflammation, tissue injury, and certain other metabolic events such as cancer. High levels are related to thrombosis (clotting) and vascular injury.

- **Histamine blood test.** Histamine is produced by basophils and by mast cells and is involved in local immune responses, as well as regulation of physiological function in the gut. In addition, histamine acts as a neurotransmitter for the brain, spinal cord, and uterus. Furthermore, histamine is involved in the inflammatory response and has a central role as a mediator of itching. It also increases the permeability of the capillaries to white blood cells and some proteins, which allows them to activate against pathogens in infected tissues. Histamine levels can also be measured in the urine and in the stool.

- **Eosinophils blood test.** Eosinophils are a type of white blood cell, and they play two roles in your immune system. They destroy foreign substances and regulate inflammation. Levels commonly elevate due to allergic reactions and parasitic and fungal infections. Levels may also rise in autoimmune disorders, skin diseases, and cancer.

- **GlycA test.** GlycA is a newer blood marker that tracks systemic inflammation and subclinical vascular inflammation.

TREATMENTS

Research is beginning to show evidence that inflammation could be a factor in a wide variety of diseases and illnesses. Fortunately, there are now conventional and Personalized Medicine remedies that present scientific promise.

CONVENTIONAL MEDICINE THERAPIES

Conventional therapies are centered on non-steroidal anti-inflammatory drugs (NSAIDs) that are both prescriptions and non-prescriptions, steroids, and second tier medications that are immune-suppressants and hydroxychloroquine.

Prescription and Non-prescription

- Hydroxychloroquine
- NSAIDs
- Steroids

Immunosuppressants.

The following are examples of this class of drugs:

- 6-mercaptopurine
- Methotrexate
- Azathioprine
- Tacrolimus
- Cyclosporine

PERSONALIZED MEDICINE THERAPIES

You don't have to rely solely on prescription and non-prescription drugs to decrease inflammation. Improving your lifestyle can balance inflammation in the body as well. It's possible to enhance your immunity the healthy way, by improving your diet and taking certain vitamins and herbal preparation. In clinical trials, furthermore, reducing alcohol intake and smoking cessation have proven effective in ameliorating inflammation and reducing the risk of cancer-related deaths.

Diet. Proper nutrition and a balanced diet can be fundamental in preventing illness, from a common cold to cancer. Dietary patterns high in refined starches, sugar, and saturated and trans-fatty acids and poor in natural antioxidants and fiber from fruits, vegetables, and whole grains, as well as poor in omega-3-fatty acids may cause an activation of the innate immune system. Most likely this is due to excessive production of proinflammatory cytokines associated with a reduced production of anti-inflammatory cytokines. Higher intake of fruit and vegetables lead to both a reduction in pro-inflammatory mediators and an enhanced immune cell profile. Avoiding the use of sugar or the intake of sugary foods and beverages can help to decrease inflammation. (See page 257 for a longer discussion on sugary foods and their role in cancer initiation and progression.)

HERBAL THERAPIES AND NUTRIENTS THAT DECREASE INFLAMMATION

The use of anti-inflammatory agents, such as aspirin, to healthy women has been associated with a reduced risk for breast cancer. Moreover, a recent meta-analysis suggested that aspirin may reduce the overall risk of breast cancer, reduce the risk of breast cancer in postmenopausal women, hormone-receptor-positive tumors, and in situ breast cancer. Without the possible side effects that exist with anti-inflammatory drugs or over-the-counter anti-inflammatory items such as aspirin, these therapies have the potential to be effective in treating or protecting against inflammation.

There are also many natural therapies that do not require a prescription to decrease inflammation in your body. Fish oil is a great anti-inflammatory supplement. Moreover, both LDN and fish oil in decreasing inflammation help to build a healthy immune system. The following are natural ways to lower inflammation in your body and to help protect yourself from many diseases including breast cancer.

American Skullcap

Skullcap may sound like the hat, but it is actually a medicinal plant that has long been used for healing purposes. This medicinal plant references two herbs: American skullcap (*scutellaria lateriflora*) and Chinese skullcap (*scutellaria baicalensis*). Each is a therapy for different medical conditions. This section refers to American skullcap (*scutellaria lateriflora*). It is a member of the mint family. American Skullcap can be taken to decrease inflammation, lower blood sugar, and for immune modulation.

Recommended dosage. The recommended dose depends on your age, kidney function, and weight.

Side effects and Contraindications. Because American skullcap can have a sedating effect, do not use it with other herbs that have a sedating effect. Also avoid taking it with any medications that have this action. Speak with your healthcare provider or pharmacist to learn if any medications you are using might make it unwise to use skullcap. High doses of American skullcap can cause any of the following symptoms: giddiness, irregular heartbeat, mental confusion, seizures, stupor, and twitching.

Berberine

Berberine is a chemical compound found in several plants, including goldenseal, Oregon grape, European barberry, and goldthread. Berberine works against infections and is anti-inflammatory. It possesses broad-spectrum therapeutic potential for various diseases such as diabetes, hypertension (high blood pressure), depression, obesity, inflammation, and cancer. The therapeutic efficacy of berberine has been reported in several studies regarding breast, colon, pancreatic, liver, oral, bone, skin, prostate, intestine, and thyroid cancers. It prevents cancer cell proliferation by inducing apoptosis (cell death) and controlling the cell cycle as well as autophagy (the breakdown of the cell that removes unnecessary components that are dysfunctional). Berberine also hinders tumor cell invasion and metastasis by down-regulating metastasis-related proteins. Moreover, this important herb is also beneficial in the early stages of cancer development by lowering epithelial–mesenchymal transition protein expression.

As previously discussed, triple-negative breast cancer (TNBC) is an aggressive breast cancer subtype. Berberine has been shown to be toxic to all treated TNBC cell lines. In addition, berberine as a potent anticancer agent significantly reduces cell viability, inhibits colony formation, cell migration, and decreases the secretion of proinflammatory cytokines (IL-1alpha, IL-6, TNF-alpha, IL-1beta).

Recommended dosage. The recommended dosage is 200 to 500 milligrams twice a day.

Side effects and Contraindications. Berberine can cause uterine contractions, so it should be avoided in pregnancy and while breastfeeding. Some drugs interfere with berberine such as cyclosporine. Speak with your healthcare provider or pharmacist to learn if any drugs you are taking may make it unwise to take this supplement. Berberine is generally safe to take. Moreover, the following digestion-related side effects may occur: constipation, cramping, diarrhea, gas, and stomach pain.

Bergamot

Bergamot has been used since the 18th century for its balsamic and medicinal properties. Bergamot juice is rich in flavonoids, including flavone and flavanone glycosides which are responsible for its beneficial effects. Numerous laboratory and human studies have demonstrated that various forms of bergamot (for example, extract, juice, essential oil, and polyphenolic fraction) can alter the functionality of several biological pathways, leading to anti-proliferative (inhibiting or slowing down the growth and division of cells) and pro-apoptotic (programed cell death) effects against cancer cells. This compound also blocked activation of stem cell-associated signaling pathways.

Recommended dosage. The recommended dosage is 500 milligrams twice a day.

Side effects and Contraindications. Increased sensitivity to sunlight: Bergamot contains compounds that can make your skin more sensitive to sunlight, potentially increasing the risk of sunburn or other skin irritation. Bergamot may interact with drugs that cause photosensitivity, as well as certain antibiotics and diabetes medications. Do not combine Bergamot with a statin drug since it may increase myopathy (muscle pain), a common side effect of statins. Some people may have allergic reactions to bergamot, resulting in a rash, itching, or difficulty breathing.

Boswellia

Boswellia (*boswellia serrata*) has been used to treat inflammatory conditions for many centuries. *Boswellia serrata* possesses monoterpenes, diterpenes, triterpenes, tetracyclic triterpenic acids and four major pentacyclic triterpenic acids which are responsible for inhibition of pro-inflammatory enzymes. It inactivates NF kappa beta (a protein complex that controls transcription of DNA, cytokine production, and cell survival) and down regulates TNF-alpha (a protein manufactured by white blood cells that when overproduced can lead to disease where the immune system acts against healthy tissues) and decreases proinflammatory cytokines.

Boswellia acts as a strong anti-inflammatory agent, lowers blood sugar, and modulates the immune system. Furthermore, it exhibits anti-cancer activity in patients with breast cancer.

Recommended dosage. The most recommended dose is to take Boswellia 300 to 500 milligrams twice a day to three times a day of an extract standardized to contain 30 to 40 percent Boswellic acids. The complete effect may take several weeks.

Side effects and Contraindications. Do not use Boswellia if you are pregnant. It may stimulate blood flow in the uterus and pelvis and therefore may increase menstrual flow and may induce miscarriage. Boswellia may also interact with NSAIDs including aspirin. Possible side effects include nausea, acid reflux, diarrhea, and skin rashes.

Chinese Skullcap

There are two forms of skullcap. This section refers to Chinese skullcap which is also known as baikal skullcap (*scutellaria baicalensis*). It is a member of the mint family. This herb has been used in China for many years to treat several health problems, including high blood pressure, hepatitis, constipation, and various viruses. In addition, it lowers your blood sugar and acts as an immune modulator, stimulating or suppressing the immune system, and may help the body fight cancer. It has also proven to be beneficial for breast cancer treatment. During chemotherapy it can decrease the risk of metastatic tumors. Chinese skullcap is particularly well known for treating conditions associated with inflammation. Its anti-inflammatory qualities are from the isoflavones it contains—baicalein, baicalin, and wogonin.

Recommended dosage. The recommended daily dose depends on your age, kidney function, and weight.

Side effects and Contraindications. Do not use Chinese skullcap with herbs that have a sedating effect: valerian, catnip, and kava. Use it with caution if you are diabetic since it lowers blood sugar. You may need less medication or other therapies for your blood sugar when taking American skullcap. This herb should not be used during pregnancy or if you are breast breast-feeding. Also, do not use Chinese skullcap if you have stomach problems or dysfunction of your spleen.

Chinese skullcap can interfere with the following medications: cyclosporine, ciprofloxacin, doxorubicin, and it may increase the risk of bleeding if you are taking warfarin. In addition, there have been reported cases of interstitial pneumonia and acute respiratory failure. This risk is increased in the elderly, with duration of usage, and if you are taking the drug interferon.

Curcumin

Curcumin is a phytonutrient derived from the spice turmeric (*Curcuma longa*) that has been used for over 4,000 years. Turmeric, the main element of curry, is a member of the ginger family. Curcumin has many medicinal benefits. It has a long history of relieving inflammation by inhibiting certain enzymes and other substances within the inflammatory pathway. It can lower LDL (bad) cholesterol and total cholesterol. Curcumin may also prove to have an anti-cancer effect. Research proposes that curcumin may prevent cancer, slow the spread, and make chemotherapy more effective, as well as shield cells from the damage caused by radiation therapy. Furthermore, clinical trials have shown that curcumin may help maintain cognition and treat inflammatory bowel diseases. It has also been shown to reduce both duodenal and gastric ulcers and used as an anti-inflammatory and to lower blood sugar.

Recommended dosage. The recommended daily dosage is 400 to 600 milligrams three times a day.

Side effects and Contraindications. If you are pregnant or breastfeeding, do not take turmeric supplements. Because curcumin may act like a blood thinner, discontinue its use two weeks before surgery. Also consult your healthcare provider before taking if you are on a drug that is a blood thinner.

Do not use it if you have gallstones since it stimulates the gallbladder to produce bile. Curcumin lowers blood sugar. If you are taking nutrients or medications for insulin resistance or diabetes, check your blood sugar on a regular basis especially if you are using this herb. Curcumin can interfere with drugs that decrease stomach acid since this herb can increase the production of stomach acid. Therefore, do not use it if you have peptic ulcers.

Fish Oil

Fish oil is a dietary source of omega-3 fatty acids and is necessary for good health. Emerging studies have shown a link in diets rich in omega-3 fatty acids with a decreased risk of breast cancer. Omega-3 fatty acids are a good source of lignans which can alter estrogen metabolism. In postmenopausal women, lignans can cause the body to process less active forms of estrogen which may potentially decrease breast cancer risks. Furthermore, your body needs omega-3 fatty acids for its anti-inflammatory effects, cell growth, lowering risks of heart disease, lowering blood pressure, and reducing blood triglyceride levels. Omega-3-fatty acids are derived from food, such as salmon, mackerel, trout, shellfish, nuts, and seeds.

Recommended dosage. The recommended dosage is 1,000 to 2,000 milligrams a day.

Side effects and Contraindications. When taken as recommended, fish oil supplements are almost always considered safe. Nevertheless, fish oil can cause a few mild side effects, such as fishy aftertaste, heartburn, nausea, diarrhea, and a rash. Consuming an overabundance of fish oil can lead to side effects such as high blood sugar and an increased risk of bleeding.

Ginger

Ginger (*Zingiber officinale*) has been used for culinary and medicinal purposes for thousands of years. The root (or rhizomes) of the ginger plant can be consumed fresh or cooked; powdered and used as a flavoring or to make tea; infused into an oil; or juiced. Medicinal forms of ginger include teas, tinctures, capsules, and lozenges. Ginger has been extensively studied and found to contain many beneficial substances. Of these, the best known are gingerols and shogaols, both of which exhibit a host of biological activities. 6-gingerol, a component of ginger, has been proven to reduce hormone receptor positive (ER-positive and PR-positive) cell growth and cell division. Additionally, 6-gingerol can kill breast cancer stem cells in the hormone receptor population. It can also balance the immune system, improve blood sugar levels, act as an antioxidant, and is an anti-inflammatory. Furthermore, it decreases your risk of developing an infection since it is antimicrobial.

Recommended dosage. The recommended dosage is 500 milligrams twice a day. Do not take more than 4 grams of ginger a day, including food sources.

Side effects and Contraindications. Ginger can act as a blood thinner. If you have a bleeding disorder or are taking a medication or supplement that may thin your blood, do not take this supplement. If you are planning to have surgery, discontinue this herbal therapy two weeks before the procedure. Speak to your healthcare provider or pharmacist to learn if any drugs you're taking might make it unwise to take ginger supplements. It is rare to have side effects from ginger, but some may occur. Taking ginger in capsule form or with meals may help you avoid the following side effects: diarrhea, heartburn, stomach upset. Used topically, ginger may cause contact dermatitis. If this occurs, discontinue use.

Green tea

Although green tea has been popular in Eastern countries, such as China, India, and Japan, for much of recorded history, it has also become increasingly popular in the Western world. Recognized for its varied medicinal benefits, green tea is particularly praised for its high content of antioxidants. It is from the Camellia sinensis plant, as are black tea and oolong tea, but is steamed rather than fermented. This allows it to retain its healthful qualities, unlike the other two teas. Green tea can be taken as a capsule or drunk as a tea.

Studies suggest that polyphenols in green tea may prevent the growth of breast cancer cells and reduce the risk of reoccurrence. The data from a study of Asian-American women cited that those women who drank more green were less likely to develop breast cancer. Women with cancer may also consume green teas because it is an antioxidant, regulates blood sugar levels, and boosts immunity. Green tea possesses one of the highest concentrations of antioxidants of any tea.

Recommended dosage. Drinking moderate amounts of green tea, up to 8 cups, is generally safe. More than 8 cups can be unsafe. Do not take directly with iron supplements since the tannins in green tea may bind to iron and decrease its absorption.

Side effects and Contraindications. Drinking great amounts may cause side effects that range from mild to serious and include:

- Avoid drinking green tea if you take blood-thinning medications.

- Green tea contains caffeine, therefore some drinkers experience insomnia or restlessness. However, the amount of caffeine contained in a glass of tea is minimal compared to that in coffee or soda.

- Some drinkers of green tea have had allergic reactions. The most common effects experienced were anxiety; constipation or diarrhea; headache; loss of appetite; and nausea.

- Due to its caffeine content, use it with caution if you have high blood pressure, cardiac arrhythmias (irregular heart rhythm), anxiety, psychiatric disorders, insomnia, or severe liver disease.

- Green tea has been shown to reduce blood levels of lithium making lithium less effective. Consult your healthcare provider if you are on lithium before drinking more than one cup of green tea a day.

- Do not use green tea if you are taking a medication that is a MAOI inhibitor.

- Caffeine from green tea, and phenylpropanolamine, used in many over the counter and prescription cough and cold medications and weight loss products, may cause mania and high blood pressure.

- Caffeinated green tea may interact negatively with several medications. Discuss this with your healthcare provider.

Pomegranate

The pomegranate (*Punica granatum L.*) is an ancient, unique fruit that grows on a small, long-living tree cultivated throughout the Mediterranean region, the Himalayas, in Southeast Asia, and in California and Arizona. The fruit of the *Punica granatum* (pomegranate) contains hundreds of phytochemicals. Pomegranate extracts have been shown to exhibit antioxidant properties, thought to be due to the action of ellagic acid, the main polyphenol in pomegranate.

The tree/fruit can be divided into several anatomical compartments: (1) seed, (2) juice, (3) peel, (4) leaf, (5) flower, (6) bark, and (7) roots, each of which has interesting pharmacologic activity. The synergistic action of the pomegranate constituents appears to be superior to that of any single component.

Pomegranate and pomegranate extracts have been reported to inhibit the spread of breast cancer and promote programmed cell death in ER positive and ER negative breast cancer cells. Specifically, pomegranate exerts antiproliferative, anti-invasive, and antimetastatic effects and induces apoptosis (cell death). It has also been shown to be beneficial in inhibiting aromatase, the conversion of testosterone to estrogen which plays an important role in breast carcinogenesis. In addition, pomegranate acts as an anti-inflammatory, antioxidant, immune modulator, aids in blood sugar regulation, and boosts immunity.

Recommended dosage. The most common dosage is 2 to 4 ounces (60 to 120 milliliters) a day. The dose is higher for hypertension: 43 to 330 milliliters of pomegranate juice a day.

Side effects and Contraindications. Generally, side effects are rare, but some people experience digestive tract symptoms, and the following may occur:

- Any medications that affect the cytochrome P450 2D6 (CYP2D6) substrates in the liver may have an interaction with pomegranate.

- Since pomegranate lowers blood pressure, one may need to decrease his or her dose of blood pressure medication.

- Do not use it if allergic to pomegranates.

- Since pomegranate affects blood pressure, discontinue use for two weeks before a scheduled surgery.

Pycnogenol

Pycnogenol is the trademarked name for a mixture of forty different antioxidants from the bark of the maritime pine tree (*Pinus maritime*). It is an oligomeric proanthocyanidin (OPC), which is one of the most common polyphenolic substances. Research acknowledges Pycnogenol for its anti-inflammatory and antioxidant properties. Studies on the use of Pycnogenol have shown anticancer activity in breast cancer cells; it has been effective in inhibiting the growth of breast cancer cells. This supplement provides a variety of health benefits, for example, improving immune function, relieving inflammation, and improving symptoms associated with menopause. It also may improve the effectiveness of Adderall in treating attention deficit disorder (ADD).

Recommended dosage. Since Pycnogenol is used for many conditions, the dosages can vary. Typical doses range from 25 to 250 milligrams a day. Take Pycnogenol with or after meals since it has an astringent taste.

Side effects and Contraindications. Side effects are rare but may include gastrointestinal discomfort, headache, nausea, and dizziness. Using Pycnogenol along with herbs and nutrients that can slow blood clotting can increase the risk of bleeding in some individuals. These herbs and nutrients include angelica, clove, garlic, nattokinase, ginger, ginkgo, Panax ginseng, vitamin E, and others. Since Pycnogenol can affect clotting time, stop using Pycnogenol at least 2 weeks before a scheduled surgery and restart two weeks after surgery. Moreover, use with caution if you have an autoimmune disease since Pycnogenol may cause the immune system to become more active.

LOW-DOSE NALTREXONE (LDN)

Personalized Medicine treatments may also include medication. Naltrexone, a non-selective antagonist of opioid receptors, is mainly used as rehabilitation therapy for discharged opiate addicts to eliminate addiction to maintain a normal life and prevent or reduce relapses. In recent years, there have been some novel and significant findings on the off-label usage of naltrexone. It is hypothesized that lower than standard doses of naltrexone (low-dose naltrexone) inhibit cellular proliferation of T and B cells and block Toll-like receptor 4 (protein coding gene), resulting in an analgesic and anti-inflammatory effect. Low-dose naltrexone is a prescription compounded medication that very effectively reduces inflammation including all forms of cancer, particularly breast cancer.

Potential short-term side effects of LDN include insomnia, vivid dreams, fatigue, loss of appetite, nausea, hair thinning, mood swing, and mild disorientation. Insomnia is the most common possible side effect which for many people resolves after the first night. Potential long-term side effects are rare and include possible liver and kidney toxicity, possible tolerance to the beneficial rebound effect. You cannot take LDN if you have acute hepatitis, liver failure, or have recent or current opioid use or if you abuse alcohol.

A few oncologists are even suggesting the use of LDN to prevent breast cancer if you have a strong family history of this disease process. LDN can reduce tumor growth by interfering with cell signaling as well as by modifying the immune system. The results of increasing studies indicate that LDN exerts its immunoregulatory activity by binding to opioid receptors in or on immune cells and tumor cells. These new discoveries indicate that LDN may become a promising agent in cancer therapy. It is an adjunct therapy and not designed to replace conventional treatment of cancer. As a daily oral therapy, LDN is inexpensive and well-tolerated.

SUMMARY

Several lines of evidence have highlighted the significance of chronic inflammation at the local and/or systemic level in breast tumor pathobiology. Inflammation can influence breast cancer progression, metastasis, and therapeutic outcome by establishing a tumor supportive immune microenvironment. These processes are mediated through a variety of cytokines and hormones that exert their biological actions either locally or throughout your entire circulation. Targeting of the immune and inflammatory pathways can be helpful not only in the development of new prevention and therapeutic strategies, but also help in better prediction of therapeutic responses in patients. Fortunately, there are many natural things that you can take to decrease inflammation. In addition, further therapies are discussed in Chapter 5 of this book concerning inflammation and the immune system. Decreasing the inflammatory response is perhaps the most important thing that you can do to decrease your risk of developing all diseases including breast cancer.

OBESITY

Obesity is defined as having too much body fat. The standard calculation is done using your Body Mass Index (BMI). If you are over your normal standard BMI, you are overweight, and over that, you are classified as obese. The proportion of adults who are obese has increased dramatically in the United States over the last 30 years. Obesity has been linked to an increased risk of developing several malignancies including a greater probability of developing breast cancer.

This association is mostly intensified in obese postmenopausal females who tend to develop estrogen-receptor-positive breast cancer. It represents a potentially controllable risk factor that you have control over. In fact, women who are lean have a lower risk of breast cancer after menopause compared to heavy women. Another study revealed the relationship between cancer risk and adult weight gain where for each 5-kilogram increase in weight, (that's a little more than 11 pounds) there was an associated 11percent increase in the risk of developing postmenopausal breast cancer.

Evidence also suggests that obesity at the time of breast cancer diagnosis is linked to an increased risk of breast cancer-specific and overall mortality in both premenopausal and postmenopausal women with early-stage breast cancer. In addition, obesity is linked to an increased risk of secondary malignancies in women with early breast cancer, and studies suggest that weight gain after diagnosis increases overall mortality. Additionally, individuals who are overweight or obese are at increased risk of developing several types of cancer. Furthermore, in a study, Wang et al. showed that females above 50 years old with greater BMI are at a greater risk of cancer compared to those with low BMI.

In other words, growing evidence from clinical studies indicates that increased adipose (body fat) is associated with increases in cancer incidence, morbidity, and mortality. Besides, the researchers observed that greater BMI is associated with more aggressive biological features of tumor, including a higher percentage of lymph node metastasis and greater size. In fact, obese women also have poorer clinical outcomes at any age including a higher probability of cancer relapse, especially in premenopausal women. Greater breast cancer risk with regards to BMI also correlates with a family history of breast cancer.

Several factors are considered to connect obesity and cancer: the insulin–IGF-1 axis, sex hormones, and the adipocyte-derived cytokines (termed adipokines—cell-signaling molecules produced by fat tissue). Each of these three factors is intimately linked to dysregulation of adipose tissue in obesity. For example, local metabolic alterations in adipose tissue in individuals with obesity result in multiple systemic metabolic alterations, such as insulin resistance, hyperglycemia (an excess of glucose in the bloodstream often associated with diabetes), dyslipidemia (high cholesterol), and chronic inflammation. Increased body fat might enhance the inflammatory state and affect the levels of circulating hormones facilitating pro-carcinogenic events.

Moreover, tumors invade stromal (connective tissue cells) compartments that are rich in adipose tissue, and adipocytes function as endocrine cells to critically shape the tumor microenvironment and contribute to tumor development and progression. In other words, these changes contribute to the increased cancer risk and poor outcomes in individuals with obesity.

Furthermore, a large body of evidence has demonstrated a significant link between obesity and cancer risk since adipose tissue and fat cells are now recognized as a highly secretory endocrine organ that produces various pro- and anti-inflammatory cytokines (proteins), estrogens, and other bioactive molecules. Likewise, obesity-related metabolic changes can influence the composition of the gut microbiome, leading to dysbiosis an imbalance between beneficial and non-beneficial bacteria which may further affect breast cancer risk and outcomes.

In addition, signaling between cancer-associated fat cells and cancer cells occurs. This crosstalk is critical for creating an environment that encourages cancer cell growth and spread. Moreover, cancer cells stimulate the breaking down of stored fat in adipocytes, which leads to removal of lipids and a fibroblast-like change in the adipocytes. These alterations in cancer-associated adipocytes are associated with functional changes in the cells, such as loss of fat-laded markers, increased secretion of inflammatory cytokines and proteases (a type of enzyme that breaks down proteins into smaller pieces), and elevated release of free fatty acids, which all support aggressive tumor growth and metastasis.

A number of recent randomized controlled trials have shown that weight loss interventions are feasible in obese survivors of breast cancer, yielding loss of five to six percent of body weight. Several ongoing randomized clinical trials are evaluating the effect of weight loss interventions on breast cancer outcomes. These studies will help define the role of weight loss in the management of obese women with early breast cancer.

KEY FACTORS THAT DRIVE OBESITY

There are four key factors for you and your healthcare provider to consider when it comes to obesity and its relationship to breast cancer. All three of these factors are blood studies that can be measured at your local laboratory or hospital.

- **Adiponectin.** Adiponectin is a protein hormone that is produced by fat cells. Its effects include the reduction of inflammation and the formation of fatty deposits in the arteries and enhancement of the response of cells to the hormone insulin which regulates your blood sugar. Strong evidence now supports an epidemiological relationship between obesity, low levels of adiponectin, and an increased incidence of breast cancer. In addition, individuals with low levels of adiponectin are up to nine times more likely to develop type 2 diabetes.

- **Hyperglycemia.** Hyperglycemia (high blood glucose) is a hallmark of both type 1 diabetes mellitus and type II diabetes. Furthermore, hyperglycemia frequently occurs in patients with other chronic diseases, such as obesity, cognitive decline, and cardiovascular disease. Furthermore, the results of clinical studies and meta-analyses indicate that an important association exists between diabetes mellitus and a subset of cancers which include liver, pancreas, endometrium, colorectal, breast, and renal cancers. Likewise, the increased prevalence of diabetes mellitus in patients with cancer has drawn attention to the effects of hyperglycemia on cancer initiation and progression. Identifying hyperglycemic conditions in individuals at the time of diagnosis could help to direct early intervention efforts towards key targets, such as HER3, in the context of breast cancer.

- **Hyperinsulinemia.** Elevated insulin levels are associated with obesity, and conversely, weight loss. If insulin does not work effectively in your body, then you will commonly gain weight. This is called insulin resistance. In order to understand insulin resistance, you have to know a little about the key role that insulin performs in the body. When you eat, your digestive system breaks food down into a type of sugar that is the body's main form of energy. The glucose is then transported through the bloodstream to cells throughout the body.

  As glucose levels rise, a signal is sent to the pancreas to create more insulin, causing blood insulin levels to rise as well. In a healthy body, the insulin then allows the sugar to move out of the bloodstream and into the cells, where it can be used. This is, in fact, insulin's most important role. It enables the body to process glucose into energy, which, in turn, fuels all the body's functions. But in the case of insulin resistance, glucose is prevented from entering the cells effectively. The pancreas reacts by producing even more insulin, but since the cells have essentially closed their doors to the glucose, the additional insulin does not do any good. Many people with insulin resistance have elevated levels of both insulin and glucose. Every time you eat, the body produces more glucose; every time your glucose levels rise, the body secretes more insulin. In some people, if insulin spikes too frequently, over time, the overworked cells become less responsive to the hormone, creating the condition known as insulin resistance.

  In fact, the newest class of drugs for weight loss called glucagon-like peptide-1 receptor agonists (GLP1-Ras) not only act by reducing weight but also can affect the mechanisms involved in insulin resistance. Insulin resistance is also commonly related to the development of breast cancer. Several studies have shown that higher insulin levels, linked to insulin resistance, are associated with an increased risk of reoccurrence and death in women with early-stage breast cancer, even in the absence of diabetes. The link between insulin resistance and breast cancer was discussed at length in the previous chapter.

- **Leptin.** Leptin is a protein produced by fat cells (adipocytes) that is a hormone acting mainly in the regulation of appetite and fat storage. Leptin receptors are expressed in almost every tissue and have a dynamic role in many organ systems, including the regulation of cancer growth. Leptin levels rise dramatically during states of obesity, and as a result, this adipokine is thought to have a pivotal role at the interface of obesity and cancer development. A meta-analysis showed that women with breast cancer frequently exhibit significantly elevated circulating levels of leptin, which suggests a role for this adipokine in disease progression.

Furthermore, patients with breast cancer who had increased levels of leptin receptor mRNA transcripts in their tumors, associated with elevated serum leptin levels, had a poorer prognosis than did their counterparts without these factors. Likewise, studies in breast cancer cell lines showed that leptin induced growth of breast tumor cells. Leptin also potently activated the migration and motility of breast cancer cells. Moreover, leptin signaling maintained cancer stem cells-like properties in triple-negative breast cancer cells (that is, lacking expression of the estrogen receptor, progesterone receptor, and HER2). Consequently, enabling cancer stem cells with self-renewal capacity to mediate tumor reoccurrence and metastasis.

Overall, these observations demonstrate that leptin-receptor signaling has a crucial role in mammary cancer progression, and that stopping this pathway would be therapeutically beneficial.

WEIGHT LOSS

Does weight loss affect cancer development and reoccurrence? The effect of weight loss on tumor initiation and progression is an important issue. In a study of 2,437 women who underwent surgical resection of early-stage breast cancer, participants who were assigned to a group with decreased dietary fat intake experienced weight loss and an improved rate of relapse-free survival compared with women in the control group.

As previously discussed, inflammation in adipose tissues (body fat) is regarded as a critical mediator of both obesity and cancer. C-reactive protein (CRP) levels, a serum marker of inflammation, are increased in individuals who are overweight or obese and decline with weight loss. In a randomized controlled trial in postmenopausal women, weight loss achieved by caloric restriction was associated with a reduction in levels of several inflammatory markers. In other words, weight loss decreased inflammation in the body, which has been shown to decrease the risk of developing breast cancer as well as lower the risk of getting the disease again. It is too early to determine if the new prescription weight loss medications discussed above, GLP1-Ras) will decrease the risk of developing breast cancer but they have been shown to decrease inflammation.

SUMMARY

The current concept that obesity is a major risk factor for development of, and mortality associated with a subset of cancers is well appreciated. As you have seen, adipose tissues that influence functions of cancer cells, such as growth, metastasis, and reoccurrence are an integral part of the tumor microenvironment. Signals between cancer-associated adipocytes and cancer cells provide an environment for the growth and metastasis of tumors.

In addition, obesity-related inflammation is a plausible link between obesity and cancer. Obesity causes low-grade chronic inflammation as well as promotes estrogen synthesis, as the aromatase enzyme synthesizes estrogens in adipose tissue from circulating androgens. Reduced levels of anti-inflammatory cytokines and increased levels of proinflammatory cytokines can have mitogenic (mitosis in cells), anti-apoptotic (prevents cell death), and angiogenic (forming new blood vessels) effects and accelerate tumor progression. Moreover, metabolic symbiosis between adipocytes and cancer cells may account, in part, for this relationship. Fortunately, the effects of obesity on cancer progression may be curbed through weight-loss intervention. If you are overweight, work with your healthcare provider to find a program that helps

CONCLUSION

Science has proven that there are several disease processes that are associated with the development of breast cancer. The health of your GI tract is so important since it is seventy percent of your immune system. Consequently, this unhealthy mycobacterial gut imbalance is linked to an increased risk of developing this form of cancer. High cholesterol, numerous kinds of infection, inflammation, and obesity are also major diseases and causes of diseases that can be treated and controlled to help decrease your risk of developing breast cancer and a reoccurrence.

8

Strengthening Your Immune System

One subject that is not commonly discussed by primary care physicians or oncologists is how your immune system works and what you can do to keep it working perfectly. An optimal immune system is a key component to help prevent breast cancer, as well as prevent a reoccurrence. This section of the book will explore how your immune system works; lifestyle changes you can make to strengthen your immunity; and herbal and nutritional therapies for immune building. Antitumor immunity is one of the body's first lines of defenses against tumors. In addition, in this section, we review the immune cells that generate an antitumor response against breast cancer.

WHAT MAKES UP YOUR IMMUNE SYSTEM?

Cells and tissues work together in harmony to form complex systems in order to serve different vital functions in your body. The immune system is one of the most crucial systems. It encompasses tissues and cells that are associated with the defense of your body from different pathogens and infectious agents, such as viruses and bacteria. The immune system is generally classified into two different types: your innate immune system, also called the *natural* immune system, and your acquired immune system, referred to as *adaptive* immunity. The purpose of both systems is to protect your body from disease or illness. In order to understand your immune system thoroughly, let us take a closer look at both of these systems in detail.

YOUR INNATE IMMUNE SYSTEM

Your innate immune system is designed to activate within minutes to hours after a foreign agent invades the body. Its purpose is to prevent the spread of harmful outside invaders. The innate immune system is composed of two lines of defense. The first line of defense consists of: the skin, mainly the epidermis or outer skin; the gastric acid in the stomach; and the mucous membranes lining the tissues that are exposed to air, such as the nasal passages. The second line of defense consists of chemicals and cells that are released in the blood after being exposed to a pathogenic stimulus. The following is a summary of the characteristics of the innate immune system:

- These cells are active since birth, are operating all the time, and are ready to perform as soon as a foreign body enters your system.

- Once activated against a specific type of antigen, a toxin, or foreign substance, this form of immunity remains in your body throughout your life.

- It is inherited from your parents and passed down to your children.

- The response recognizes all types of pathogens, including viruses, bacteria, and fungi.

- The same response is produced every time a pathogen invades the body.

- Its ability to fight off certain pathogens is limited.

YOUR ADAPTIVE IMMUNE SYSTEM

The adaptive system is mainly responsible for more complex reactions. This system activates after the innate response is fully implemented. Initially, the antigen entering the body is identified by the specific immune cells. Then a cascade of reactions is started in the form of an antigen-antibody reaction to attack these outside invaders. This immune system also has the ability to remember these antigens, so that a specific response will be started should the same pathogen enter your body again in the future. The following is a summary of the characteristics of the adaptive immune system:

- These cells are normally in silent mode and become active only when the antigen is identified.

- The response is not immediate. It may begin to appear a week or two after it has identified the outside invader. Consequently, it is called a delayed response type of immunity.

- The potency and effectiveness levels are very high, since the combat cells the body generates are greatly specialized and also very powerful.

- The span of developed immunity may last for a short time—or a lifetime.

- Unlike the cells of the innate immune system, these cells are not inherited.

- Each of these cells has a very specific purpose.

- Memory cells are present, which identifies specific cells on each exposure.

- This immunity system has the ability to recognize and respond to a wide range of outside invaders.

Despite the differences, both immune systems have the same overall function—to protect you from harm. The innate response is produced initially for complete elimination of the pathogen, and then the delayed response is produced in the form of adaptive immunity—to continue to fight the battle and remember the identity of the invading enemy. Cells of both the systems coordinate equally to produce an effective and long-lasting response, protecting us against harmful pathogens and infectious agents from entering the body. Furthermore, there are both similarities and differences between the cells produced by the innate and adaptive immune classifications.

CELLS OF THE INNATE AND ADAPTIVE IMMUNE SYSTEMS

The cells of both the innate and adaptive immune systems originate in the bone marrow, which produces hematopoietic stem cells; that is, the cells that generate other blood cells. These stem cells then change into two cell lines.

▧ Myeloid Stem Cells (Innate)

These myeloid stem cells can change into the red blood cells, platelets, neutrophils, eosinophils, basophils, and monocytes. The monocytes then make the dendritic cells and the macrophages. *These are the cells that comprise\your innate immune system.*

- **Dendritic cells.** These cells activate other immune cells by identifying antigens to other cells.

- **Phagocytic cells.** These cells engulf and attack potential threats, like viruses and bacteria. Phagocytic cells include basophils, eosinophils, macrophages, monocytes, and neutrophils.

- **Epithelial and endothelial cells.** These are cells that line the respiratory, gastrointestinal, and genitourinary tracts, acting as a protective shield against pathogens.

- **Granulocytes.** A type of white blood cell that primarily fights bacterial and fungal infections by releasing granules that contain enzymes designed to kill pathogens.

- **Mast cells.** These are a type of white cell that releases histamines that signal other cells to produce chemicals to counteract the effects of pathogens.

- **Basophils.** Also a type of white blood cell that contains granules filled with histamine, which is released when they encounter allergens.

■ Lymphoid Stem Cells (Adaptive)

Such cells give rise to natural killer cells, T lymphocytes, and B lymphocytes. *This is your adaptive immune system.* In addition, these cells also make other cells.

- **Natural killer (NK) cells.** These are another type of white blood cell. They are an important component of the innate immune system. They identify and attack cells that are abnormal, infected, and/or diseased, such as tumor cells.

- **B lymphocytes (B cells).** A type of white blood cell that produces antibodies that attach to and attack pathogens.

- **T lymphocytes (T cells).** A type of white blood cell that produces *cytokines*, which are biological substances that activate other parts of the immune system.

CYTOKINES

Cytokines are small proteins that act as messengers to help regulate the immune response and communication between cells. They can signal cells to help control inflammation in your body. They are crucial in controlling the growth and activity of other immune system cells and blood cells. They allow your immune system to mount a defense against microbes that enter your body.

Adverse effects of cytokines have been linked to many disease processes, such as schizophrenia, depression, most forms of cancer (including breast cancer), and Alzheimer's disease. The exact initiation process of breast cancer is unknown, although several hypotheses theories have emerged. Inflammation has been proposed as an important player in tumor initiation, promotion, angiogenesis, and metastasis, all phenomena in which cytokines are prominent players. Data suggests that cytokines play an important role in the regulation of both induction and protection in breast cancer. This knowledge could be fundamental for the proposal of new therapeutic approaches to breast cancer and other cancer-related disorders. Oversecretion of cytokines can trigger a cytokine storm.

Cytokine Storm

Under normal circumstances, cytokines help coordinate the response of your immune system to take care of infectious substances, like viruses or bacteria. The problem is that sometimes the body's inflammatory response can get out of control, causing more harm than good. From time to time, the body produces too many inflammatory cytokines, which promote inflammation, and not enough cytokines that regulate inflammation. Consequently, the inflammatory cytokines start "storming" out of control, without enough feedback from the anti-inflammatory cytokines.

Recent studies have shown that in people experiencing cytokine storm syndrome, certain cytokines are present in the blood at higher-than-normal amounts, which can cause multisystem organ failure and even death.

Cytokine storms can be triggered by several infectious and non-infectious causes including certain autoimmune conditions, pathogens, various therapies, viruses, and cancer treatments. Cytokine storm can cause the same kind of symptoms that an infection would. One may experience flu-like and respiratory symptoms, body aches, high fevers, and, in general, not feeling well. Sometimes the symptoms are only mild but at other times, they can be severe and life-threatening.

HUMORAL AND CELL-MEDIATED IMMUNITY

The adaptive system can further be divided into two categories: *humoral immunity* and *cell-mediated* immunity.

What are the similarities between humoral and cell-mediated immunity?

- Humoral and cell-mediated immunity are two types of adaptive immunity.

- Both immunity types activate upon the exposure to foreign antigens.

- They effectively defend your body against a variety of pathogens.

- Each of the immunities creates immunological memory against antigens.

- The mutual systems do not work correctly in immune-compromised individuals.

What are the differences between humoral and cell-mediated immunity?

- Humoral immunity relies on the production of antibodies by B cells (which uses body fluids to fight pathogens), while cell-mediated immunity involves T cells that go directly after infected cells.

IMMUNE SYSTEM AND BREAST CANCER

A strong immune system will play a crucial role in preventing the development of breast cancer, as well as its progression. If you have already had breast cancer, strengthening your immune system will help prevent a reoccurrence. In addition, current treatments for breast cancer include surgical intervention, radiotherapy, chemotherapy, and hormone replacement therapy (HRT). These are usually applied to non-invasive or non-metastatic breast cancers. Immunotherapy is one promising approach to address invasive and metastatic breast cancers. Using immune cells as a treatment can help the body recognize and target cancer cells. There are multiple different techniques for immunotherapy.

Adoptive cell therapy is a branch of cancer immunotherapy that utilizes the immune cells to attack cancer cells. One of the first methods of immunotherapy created was cytokine therapy, which uses cytokines to activate certain immune cells to antitumor immunity. In addition, as you have seen, natural killer (NK) cells are an essential component of innate immunity and are critical in destroying tumor cells without prior stimulation with antigens.

SUMMARY

The predominant function of the immune system is to prevent or regulate infection. The immune system is complex and extensive, with a myriad of cell types that flow throughout your body performing a unique role. Each of the cell types has distinct ways of identifying problems, communicating with other cells, and carrying out their functions. When scientists better understand the workings of these cells, it allows them to confront specific health problems, extending their treatments from infections to cancer.

Certain breast cancer treatments, such as chemotherapy, can weaken the immune system. Therefore, maintaining a strong immune system is paramount. Eating healthily, exercise, getting enough sleep, and reducing stress can help to boost your immune system.

HOW IS YOUR IMMUNE SYSTEM MEASURED?

Laboratory studies are essential to determine the presence of a primary immunodeficiency disease. These tests are generally ordered by a physician when an individual experiences some type of inflammatory problem.

Standard blood tests can determine if you have normal levels of infection-fighting proteins called *immunoglobulins* in your blood. If you have too few immunoglobulins in your body, it gives you a greater chance of getting infections, autoimmune diseases, or certain forms of cancer. Having too many may mean you may have allergies, or an autoimmune disorder. It may also indicate that something else in your body may be triggering such a response.

FACTORS THAT AFFECT YOUR IMMUNE SYSTEM

Most of us never really think about our immune systems. They carry on their jobs of protecting us in silence. The only way we may become conscious of them is when they are needed to fight an infection; or if the results of a blood test indicate we may have a health problem. Few of us spend much time thinking about the protection it provides until we have a problem. By understanding what influences our immune systems, we are in a better position to protect ourselves. To begin with, let's look at the major factors that play a significant role in how strong or weak your immune system is.

■ INFLUENCE OF AGING

As you age, your immune system ages as well. This process is called *immunosenescence*. It becomes evident that there is an increasing deterioration in your capacity to respond to vaccines efficiently. Because of this, you are more likely to get sick and to recuperate from injuries, infection, and disorders at a slower pace. Since there is no predetermined age when immunity decreases, it is crucial to go to the doctor routinely and get medical support if you get sick frequently or if you're having difficulty healing after injury or illness. Research has shown that a decline in immune function is the most recognized effect of aging, which is associated with an increased risk in developing breast cancer (as seen in Part 1 of this book).

Immunity also becomes imbalanced in old age. This affects the two branches of the immune system, the innate immunity and adaptive immunity. With age, many individuals do not show signs and symptoms of their infection or disease process, which leads to a possible issue with expedient diagnosis and treatment. Likewise, as you age, changes in the immune system can occur. There are fewer immune cells in the body to prompt healing, which results in a slower healing process.

The immune system's ability to recognize and correct cell defects also decreases, in addition to a decline in tissue renewal capability that can result in an increased risk of cancer. Since breast cancer can be an age-related disease, the influence of aging on tumor immune responses may have crucial consequences. Today, the rate of breast cancer has shown to increase with age, from 1.5 cases per 100,000 in women ages 20 to 24 to a peak of over 400 cases per 100,000 in women ages 75 to 79. In fact, ninety-five percent of new cases of breast cancer occur in women over the age of 40, which may be due to the body's decline in immune health that occurs with age.

■ INFLUENCE OF STRESS

In addition, as your immune system weakens, it may be significantly influenced by psychological stress and related stress hormones. In fact, there are similarities between a weakened immune system and stress-related immunological changes.

Likewise, chronic stress during aging leads to accelerated immune weakness for both the patient and their caretaker. Markers of inflammation, such as IL-6 and c-reactive protein (CRP), may increase as well as NF-kB (which is an important pro-inflammatory transcription factor). Consequently, chronic stress has been shown to lead to premature aging of the T cells of the immune system. Moreover, a history of stressful life events has been found to be associated with a moderate increase in the risk of developing breast cancer.

■ INFLUENCE OF ENVIRONMENTAL AND LIFESTYLE FACTORS

As you have seen, immune weakness is characterized by its high prevalence, individual variability, and complexity. In other words, the immune system is not uniformly affected by the aging process. New studies suggest that part of this personalized immune response that occurs with aging is weakness in your immune system—it is not only the result of aging, but rather is also due to secondary changes caused by environmental and lifestyle factors. Exposure to environmental pollutants and toxic chemicals are risks for breast cancer, especially as you age. Recently, however, new cases of breast cancer have been occurring more commonly in younger women (which may be due to the toxic load they are carrying from the environment that also compromises their immunity).

Older women who are physically inactive or overweight also have a higher risk of getting breast cancer. Nutrition, exercise, and even medications taken during your life can influence immune function with age.

SUMMARY

While people are living longer, the increase in longevity does not always coincide with the increase in *healthspan*—the healthy years in one's living a quality of life. As a way of counteracting the effects of a decline in the immune system, healthcare providers may recommend a comprehensive healthy eating program, exercise, vitamins and herbal supplements, hormone replacement therapy, and improvement of gut health. Tips on living a healthy lifestyle, and herbal and nutritional therapies, to help build your immune system to prevent breast cancer and a reoccurrence are discussed in the remainder of this section of the text.

LIFESTYLE CHANGES TO STRENGTHEN YOUR IMMUNITY

Let us now examine lifestyle changes that can strengthen your immunity. Most of these ten key strategies you can use on your own without a healthcare provider's input. It is always best, however, to keep your doctor or other health professional updated on changes in diet, nutrients, and other things that you are doing to help heal and build your immune system.

This section covers ten key strategies to help prevent breast cancer and, if you have already had this disease, to prevent it from coming back or spreading.

- **Alcohol**: Moderation or Abstinence is the Key to Good Health

- **Exercise**: Whether You Like It or Not

- **Gut**: A Healthy Gut Equals a Healthy Immune System

- **Inflammation**: Its Effect on Your Immune System

- **Sleep**: Get a Good Night's Sleep

- **Smoking**: How It Affects the Immune System

- **Stress**: Manage Your Stress

- **Sugar**: Minimize Your Intake

- **Thyroid**: Optimize Its Function

- **Water**: Stay Hydrated

The following sections will help you understand ways to maximize your immune system and help balance the functions in your body so that it performs optimally as well as decreasing your risk of developing breast cancer, discouraging the spread of breast cancer, and hopefully stopping it from happening again. As you will notice, many of these key components are the same ones that are risk factors for the development of breast cancer (as described and explored earlier in this book across Chapters 4, 5, 6, and 7). Consequently, this chapter will go further into depth on these previously-introduced subjects.

■ ALCOHOL—MODERATION, OR ABSTINENCE, IS THE KEY TO HEALTH

As you saw in the previous chapter on modifiable risk factors for breast cancer, alcohol intake is a risk factor for breast cancer. Excessive alcohol ingestion can also compromise your immune system. Some people can enjoy moderate amounts of alcohol, a glass of wine with food and drink in social settings, without any problems. However, as you will see, there is conflicting data regarding mild consumption of alcohol and your health. Even though millions of Americans, on average, consume 10 to 11 drinks weekly, many people don't appreciate the degree to which it may harm your body. Excessive drinking, which includes binge drinking and especially *heavy* drinking, can take a heavy toll on your physical (as well as mental) health in the long run. Alcohol abuse can negatively influence multiple pathways of the immune response, leading to an increased risk of developing infections. The course and resolution of both bacterial and viral infections are severely impaired in alcohol-abusing individuals, which also results in greater morbidity and mortality.

Effects on the Immune System

Immediate and chronic alcohol use has major immune effects on the body. Cells of the innate immune system are weakened by alcohol in their capacity to respond to pathogens that present to your body. In addition, inflammatory cell responses (including production of pro-inflammatory cytokines) are inhibited by acute alcohol exposure, while chronic use of alcohol increases these pro-inflammatory responses. Likewise, the antigen-presenting function of both monocytes and dendritic cells is impaired by both acute and chronic alcohol use—and this contributes to impaired production of adaptive immune responses. In addition, both acute (immediate) and chronic use of alcohol negatively impacts both T and B cell function.

■ ALCOHOL AND CANCER

As specified by the American Cancer Society (ACS), there may be a direct link between alcohol use and many types of cancer (including breast cancer).

In addition, alcohol alters the composition of your gut microbiome; and by damaging those cells, you decrease your body's defense mechanism. Consuming even small amounts of alcohol (about one drink a day) is linked with an increased risk of breast cancer in women. One study revealed that as low as three to six drinks per week increased the risk of developing this disease. Alcohol can increase levels of estrogen and other hormones that are associated with breast cancer. It may also cause unwanted weight gain, which can lead to an increased risk of cancer. Moreover, evidence shows that possible early indicators of risk, such as benign breast disease and increased breast density, are associated with alcohol consumption.

Moderation is the key to health, unless you have breast cancer on both sides of your family. If you do, then the American Cancer Society recommends that you *abstain* from alcohol use. One of the reasons is not just that alcohol increases your risk of breast cancer by elevating estrogen levels in your body, but excessive drinking compromises your immune system since it alters cytokine balance, and it is associated with decreased lymphocytes and an increased risk of developing both bacterial and viral infections.

SUMMARY

As science has shown, too much alcohol can have many devastating effects on your health. One of the least-appreciated medical complications of alcohol abuse is altered immune regulation, leading to immunodeficiency and autoimmunity (the immune system acts against its own tissues). The consequences of immunodeficiency include increased susceptibility to bacterial pneumonia, tuberculosis, and other infectious diseases as well as cancer, particularly breast cancer. Moderation or abstinence of alcohol intake is the key to health, depending on your family history.

EXERCISE—WHETHER YOU LIKE IT OR NOT

Disciplined, consistent exercise is linked to significant benefits in your overall immune system health. The body's defense against infections (as you have seen earlier in this text) is a modifiable risk factor for the development of breast cancer. In the short term, exercise aids the immune system in detecting and tackling viruses and bacteria; in fact, lack of activity is an independent risk factor for more than twenty-five chronic diseases. Over the long term, regular exercise decelerates the changes that occur to the immune system.

Regarding the direct effect on the immune system, moderate exercise seems to exert a protective effect whereas repeated bouts of *strenuous* exercise can result in compromised immune function (along with an elevation in the stress hormone cortisol and the neurotransmitter epinephrine). Consequently, exercise in moderation is one of the keys to a healthy immune system. True exercise is defined as doubling your pulse for twenty (20) minutes.

This section will discuss the effects that exercise has on the immune system in relation to lack of exercise, the right amount of exercise, vigorous exercise, and *very* vigorous exercise programs. Regular physical activity exerts a multitude of beneficial health effects but, perhaps more importantly, is its ability to both enhance immune defense and mitigate the deleterious effects of stress on immunity.

The fact of the matter is that we live in an increasingly sedentary society, since modern technology and longer hours at desk jobs (whether at home or in the workplace) have made it less necessary (and less convenient) to be physically active. The annual National Health Interview Survey found that only 35 percent of adults over the age of eighteen engage in some kind of physical activity on a regular basis. A staggering one-third of adults do not engage in any activity at all. These statistics reflect the alarming—and rising—rates of obesity, diabetes, and heart disease in the United States and all developing nations, not to mention high blood pressure, elevated cholesterol levels, and change in immune function.

WHAT IS EXERCISE?

There is an important distinction between physical activity and exercise. Physical activity is a general term that can be applied to any movement that engages the muscles, ranging from daily chores such as gardening, making beds, or vacuuming, to rigorous sports like tennis, running, or swimming, which raise the heart rate and build endurance. The term exercise, however, refers to planned, purposeful movement specifically intended to boost physical fitness. Running, walking, biking, swimming, sports, hot yoga, and dancing are all activities that require effort, expend energy, and work core muscle groups.

BENEFITS OF EXERCISE

Regular exercise is one of the most vital tasks for your well-being and good health, your body and mind. You can experience the health benefits of exercise, regardless of age, sex, physical abilities, ethnicity, shape, or size. Exercise can lessen your risk of developing breast cancer. Physical activity lowers blood estrogen levels, and women with lower blood estrogen levels have a reduced risk of breast cancer than those with too high a level. Exercise can reduce the risk of the cancer's reoccurrence and may ease the side effects associated with treatments.

Exercise provides other benefits that may help decrease the risks of breast cancer, such as an anti-inflammatory influence, enhancement of the immune system, promotion of weight loss, the lowering of elevated blood sugar, and improvement of sleep, to name a few.

Exercise has a variable effect on the immune system. If you do not exercise or only exercise occasionally, your immune system may be compromised. If you exercise the right amount, it builds your immune system; and if you exercise vigorously daily it can compromise your immune system.

HOW EXERCISE IMPROVES YOUR IMMUNE SYSTEM

Exercise in the short term helps the immune system to locate and control foreign invaders; and in the long term, it decelerates the changes that occur to the immune system with aging. The immune system benefits from exercise due to frequent mobilization and redistribution of effector lymphocytes, white blood cells—natural killer cells, T cells, and B cells. Billions of lymphocytes are mobilized in response to a single bout of exercise. Virus-specific memory T cells mobilized with exercise exhibit enhanced proliferation responses to viral antigens, common viruses that cause a range of illnesses (cold-like symptoms, fever, sore throat, pneumonia). This process is also vital to minimize the impact of the virus and to expedite viral resolution should your immune barriers be breached and you become infected.

Exercise also releases various cytokines (interferon, interleukin) from the skeletal muscle. In fact, in order to help boost immunity and mitigate the harmful effects of inactivity and social isolation stress on our immune system, it is imperative that you strive to maintain recommended exercise levels in times of increased infection rate, such as the COVID-19 pandemic.

The Physical Activity Guidelines for Americans recommend 150 to 300 minutes of moderate to vigorous intensity cardiorespiratory physical activity per week and two sessions per week of muscle-strength training. This may be more challenging if you do not have access to gyms and parks and follow social distancing and hygienic guidelines. There are many creative ways to stay vigorous at home, nevertheless. As we have seen during the COVID-19 pandemic, increased home-based exercise, such as online instructor-led classes, are useful for some people. However, specialized equipment is not required; keeping active indoors or outdoors through activities such as walking and gardening can also be beneficial. This includes my personal favorite form of exercise, which is dancing.

MODERATE-TO-VIGOROUS EXERCISE

Acute exercise (moderate-to-vigorous intensity, less than 60 min) is now viewed as an important immune system support to stimulate the ongoing exchange of distinct and highly active immune cell subtypes between the circulation and tissues. In particular, each exercise routine improves the anti-pathogen activity which has an additive effect to enhance immune defense activity and metabolic health.

The most important finding that has emerged from exercise immunology studies is that positive immune changes take place during each bout of moderate physical activity. This is consistent with public health guidelines urging individuals to engage in routine physical activity of 30 minutes or more. There is a general consensus that regular bouts of short-lasting (up to 45 minutes), moderate-intensity exercise is beneficial for host immune defense, particularly in older adults and people with chronic diseases.

- **Vigorous exercise program.** In contrast, the infection rate is reported to be higher among extreme performance athletes and is second only to injury for the number of training days lost during preparation for major events. Numerous studies, over the last 35 years, report an increase in upper respiratory infection (URI) symptoms in athletes during periods of heavy training and competition. Both innate and acquired immunity are often reported to decrease transiently in the hours after heavy exertion, typically 15 to 70 percent. In fact, prolonged heavy training sessions have been shown to decrease immune function which may provide an opportunity for infections to take hold.

- **How aggressive exercise may positively affect your immune system.** Since exercise increases blood flow as your muscles contract, it also increases the circulation of immune cells. In cranking up your circulation, it has been found to reduce stress, have drug-like effects that may alter the cross-talk unwanted signals between the immune system and tumorigenesis—formation of tumors. For example, exercise may play a role in a role in antitumor response and decrease inflammatory influences that support cancer cell growth.

- **Nutritional replenishment for vigorous exercise.** The risk of infection is increased if the individual's nutritional status is not optimal, particularly if heavy exertion lasts longer than 90 minutes. Vigorous exercise depletes the body of important nutrients, such as coenzyme q-10 and alpha-lipoic acid. Taking 300 mg a day of each of these nutrients will help replenish the mitochondria that becomes depleted during a rigorous exercise program.

- **Exercise delays the onset of the immunosenescence system for older adults.** Therefore, exercise can improve the immune system in individuals over the age of 65, which are a group of people where the immune system has shown a significant decline due to the aging process.

EXERCISE AND THE GUT MICROBIOTA

Lastly, your gut bacteria composition and diversity are influenced by a variety of factors, including dietary and exercise habits, age, genetics, ethnicity, antibiotics, health, and disease. Even weight affects this relationship. Your health of your GI tract is the biggest determinant of your immune system. (See the section that follows for a longer discussion on this important topic.)

SUMMARY

As you have seen, there are many ways to improve your immune system; however, *moderation* is the key to health. Too little exercise or too vigorous an exercise program can compromise the immune system. A planned, well-thought out, moderate exercise program is one of the main recipes for building and enhancing your immune system.

In addition, exercise may help rejuvenate the aging immune system by delaying the onset of immunological aging or even rejuvenating aged immune profiles. There is also increasing evidence that exercise training has a summation effect over time in modulating tumor growth, atherosclerosis, and other disease processes along with immune building.

THE GUT: A HEALTHY GUT EQUALS A HEALTHY IMMUNE SYSTEM

You are what you eat! Triggers, such as a poor diet, can lead to gastrointestinal (GI) challenges and gastrointestinal imbalances, which have been identified as a factor in many immune and autoimmune conditions. Recent research certainly supports this statement. Growing evidence also supports the concept that the microbiota plays a significant role in maintaining nutritional, metabolic, and immunologic homeostasis in the host. In addition, the microbiota not only maintains gastrointestinal balance but also exerts metabolic functions in nutrient digestion and absorption, detoxification, and vitamin production. Importantly, one of the principal regulators of circulating estrogens is the gut microbiome. Studies have also shown that there is a gut-mammary connection. Consequently, to prevent breast cancer, and also decrease your risk of developing breast cancer in the future, as well as a reoccurrence, it is paramount that your gut be healthy.

As you read this part of the book, it is important to understand two terms that sometimes are used interchangeably; however, they do not really mean the same thing. Human *microbiota* is the term used to describe all the specific microorganisms (bacteria, eukaryotes, archaea, and viruses) that reside within the human body; in other words, the community of microorganisms themselves. The *microbiome* represents the broader ecosystems in which these microorganisms exist. This includes not only the microbiota, but also the genes, proteins, metabolites, and all other factors that interact with these microorganisms.

This part of the book explores metabolic approaches to gastrointestinal (GI) imbalance. The regulatory control of digestion and absorption are under strict management of the neuronal and hormonal systems, and there are many causes of digestion and absorption problems. Some are due to mechanical issues, such as mastication, motility, and permeability. Likewise, GI complaints are due to multifactorial dysfunctions. Inability to digest effectively may lead to bloating, gas indigestion, constipation, diarrhea, and/or abdominal complaints.

Abnormal permeability of the intestinal wall can lead to leaky gut syndrome, yeast overgrowth, development of food allergies, and toxin production. Low gastric acidity can lead to symptoms of bloating, belching, burning, and flatulence immediately after ingesting a meal. A deficiency of gastric enzymes may lead to delayed breakdown of protein and result in symptoms of protein maldigestion. Likewise, pancreatic enzymes are required to break proteins into peptides, and a deficiency of proteolytic enzymes (produced by the pancreas and stomach) is another reason that the digestion of protein by the body may not work optimally.

Therapeutic approaches to restoration of enzymatic function—and to reduce inflammation—are key components that are addressed in this section. Food triggers, such as allergies to gluten and dairy, will also be examined. You will learn how to optimize the health of your gut through the "5R" program of **R**emove, **R**eplace, **R**epopulate, **R**epair, and **R**ebalance (already first discussed, as is much of what you will read across the next various sections, in Chapter 7, "Controllable Health Disorder Risk Factors," on page 162).

THE GASTROINTESTINAL TRACT

Your gastrointestinal tract (GI tract) is literally 70 percent (70%) of your immune system. In the GI tract can be found the largest blood supply in the body using one-third of the total blood flow from the heart. The gut flora contains 400 different microbial species. Consequently, the gut has a massive amount of influence on your metabolism. It is really a hidden organ! It has greater metabolic activity than the liver, with ten times the number of cells and 100 times the genomic material. The cells of the intestinal tract are shed and replaced every three to six days. Therefore, they are very sensitive to nutrition and lifestyle choices.

Function of the GI Tract

Therefore, if your gut is not healthy—then *you* are not healthy. The question remains: What does the GI tract actually *do* in the body? It is responsible for digestion, absorption, and detoxification of pesticides and other toxins along with eliminating 25 percent of the estrogen that your body makes or is taken as a medication. The gut also helps eliminate items that are digested and detoxified along with exclusion, which keeps substances from entering the body.

GI Microbiome and the GI Barrier

How do you have a healthy gut? From a traditional medicine viewpoint, you have a healthy GI tract when you have met these five major criteria: *effective digestion and absorption of food, absence of GI illness, normal and stable intestinal microbiota, effective immune status,* and *status of well-being.* There is now ample evidence that two functional entities are also key to achieving and maintaining gut health. These entities are the GI microbiome and the GI barrier, which is not just a mechanical barrier assessed by permeability measurements.

Multiple functions of the GI microbiome have been described. The GI microbiome prevents colonization by potentially pathogenic microorganisms, provides energy for the gut wall from undigested food, and regulates the mucosal immune system. Most importantly, the GI microbiota contributes to the maintenance of an intact GI barrier, which is closely related to infectious, inflammatory, and allergic diseases.

The *gastrointestinal mucosa*—membrane rich in mucus—forms a barrier between the body and potential hostile microorganisms and toxins. In addition, the GI barrier allows the stomach to safely store the gastric acid that is necessary for digestion.

INTESTINAL DYSFUNCTION

As mentioned in Chapter 7, almost half of the adults in the US experience intestinal illness at some time in their lives. Even emotional trauma can negatively impact your digestion. The following are signs of poor digestion and then optimal digestion, and it may surprise you that to have perfect digestion, one should ideally have two normal bowel movements a day.

Signs of Poor Digestion

☐ Chronic indigestion after eating

☐ Chronically coated tongue

☐ Depressed without a reason

☐ Feeling better if you do *not* eat

☐ Feeling stress without a cause

☐ Foul-smelling stools

☐ Frequent burping, passing gas, and/or bloated stomach

☐ Frequently cold for no reason

☐ Increase in pulse of 20 to 25 beats within 15 minutes after eating

☐ Less than one bowel movement a day

☐ Needing to loosen your belt after eating (even if you did not overeat)

☐ Poor sleeping habits/waking up tired

☐ Undigested food in stools

Signs of Optimal Digestion

☐ Do not have frequent mood swings, shakiness, anxiety, or depression without a reason

☐ Feeling better after exercising

☐ Feeling good after eating (and several hours later)

☐ Good energy level throughout the day

☐ No extreme food cravings

☐ No undigested food in stools

☐ Sleeping well (and waking up rested)

☐ Stools do not smell

☐ Two bowel movements a day

☐ Warm extremities

The GI tract needs basic nutrients: B vitamins, such as B_1, B_6; folic acid; and also vitamins A, C, D, and E. The gut also needs minerals, such as zinc, selenium, manganese, molybdenum, magnesium, and the amino acid arginine. Therefore, starting with a good multivitamin that is pharmaceutical-grade is a great place to start your journey to optimal GI health.

DYSBIOSIS (IMBALANCE IN THE GUT)

As first discussed earlier in Chapter 7, *dysbiosis* is an inflammatory disease of the GI tract due to imbalance of intestinal bacteria. The consequences of dysbiosis are great, including loss of good bacteria and loss of the production of some important vitamins. In addition, the gastrointestinal tract is one of the body's five organs of detoxification. Consequently, if you have dysbiosis, your body does not detoxify well. Furthermore, dysbiosis can cause you to lose protection from chemical toxins and antibiotics (along with having a subsequent overgrowth of harmful bacteria). Recent studies indicate that dysbiosis increases your risk of developing breast cancer.

Symptoms of Dysbiosis

Many symptoms can occur due to dysbiosis, including ones that are related to both inside and outside the GI tract, and extraintestinal symptoms.

Common symptoms include:

- Abdominal distention and bloating
- Abdominal pain
- Altered bowel function (constipation and/or diarrhea)
- Belching
- Bloating
- Cramping
- Cramps and spasms
- Flatulence
- Halitosis
- Heartburn
- Hypersecretion of colonic
- Mucus
- Nausea

Extraintestinal symptoms linked to dysbiosis include:

- Anxiety
- Brain fog
- Cognitive and memory deficit
- Depression
- Fatigue
- Fever of unknown origin
- Frequent urination
- Joint pain
- Inflammation in the vein
- Itching
- Malaise
- Muscle pain
- Palpitations
- Seizures
- Skin rashes
- Vasculitis

Causes of Dysbiosis

The causes of dysbiosis are numerous. Consequently, it is a common problem. It is often due to one, or a combination, of the following:

- Activate neutrophils caused by the escape of bacteria and large molecules of undigested food through the compromised intestinal barrier

- Alcohol abuse

- Artificial sweeteners cause glucose intolerance by altering the gut microbiota and induce dysbiosis

- Breakdown intercellular integrity

- Carbohydrate malabsorption

- Consumption of infected foods

- Corticosteroid use

- Damage the mitochondria (turn energy from food into energy the cell can use)

- Damage the mucosal lining

- Diminished bile

- Ethanol and acetaldehyde (one of the breakdown products of ethanol) disrupt the tight junctions in the cells lining the intestines which increases membrane permeability.

- Excessive stress

- Food allergies and sensitivities

- Free radical production

- Gastrointestinal surgeries

- Hypoxia/exposure to extreme altitude

- Immune deficiencies

- Improper fasting or dieting

- Lectins are protein fragments of foods that are not completely digested that bind with specific sugars on the surface cells throughout the body. They stick to the lining of the GI tract, which causes inflammation and can destroy cell membranes. Lectins flatten the intestinal villi and consequently decrease the absorption of nutrients.

- Low levels of hydrochloric acid in the stomach

- Nutritional deficiencies

- Pancreatic insufficiency

- Recirculated waste products from the liver

- Repeated use of antibiotics

- Travel

- Use of non-steroidal anti-inflammatory drugs (NSAIDs)

- Viruses like rotaviruses have proteins on their outer surfaces that can open the cellular spaces between the tight junctions of the GI mucous cells

- Yeast infections

SMALL INTESTINAL BOWEL OVERGROWTH (SIBO)

As previously mentioned, the human intestinal microbiota is composed of trillions of cells, including bacteria, viruses, and fungi and it creates a complex polymicrobial ecology—a presence of several species. This is characterized by its high population density, as well as wide diversity and complexity of interaction. An imbalance of this complex intestinal microbiome, both qualitative and quantitative, may have serious health consequences for the body, including small intestinal bowel overgrowth, commonly called SIBO. It is a specific *kind* of dysbiosis.

In other words, the GI tract is full of bacteria, it just had to be the right kind of bacteria and the right number of bacteria. SIBO is defined as an increase in the number and/or alteration in the type of bacteria in the upper gastrointestinal tract, where it does not belong. This overgrowth of bacteria usually only occurs in the colon, which is the large intestine. The body has mechanisms for preventing bacterial overgrowth: gastric acid secretion, intestinal motility, intact ileocecal valve, immunoglobulins within intestinal secretion, and bacteriostatic properties of pancreatic and biliary secretion. In some people, more than one cause may be involved in the development of SIBO.

Symptoms

Symptoms related to SIBO are:

☐ Abdominal pain   ☐ Diarrhea   ☐ Malnutrition

☐ Bloating   ☐ Malabsorption   ☐ Weight loss

The diagnosis is made by an upper GI aspirate or three-hour lactulose breath test for hydrogen/methane.

Causes

SIBO is commonly the cause of a (motility) movement problem in the small intestine. If something impairs movement, such as one or more of the following, the small intestine is unable to properly eliminate the bacteria:

- Achlorhydria (low stomach acid)

- Excessive use of antibiotics

- Gastrointestinal conditions (irritable bowel syndrome, inflammatory bowel disease, and celiac disease)

- History of bowel surgeries or anatomical abnormalities (small intestinal obstruction, diverticula, fistulae, surgical blind loop, previous ileocecal resections)

- Immunodeficiency syndromes

- Impaired valve separating the small and large intestines (ileocecal valve)

- Long-term use of proton pump inhibitors (PPIs)

- Motility disorders (scleroderma, autonomic neuropathy in diabetes mellitus, post-radiation enteropathy, small intestinal pseudo-obstruction)

- Pancreatic exocrine insufficiency

- Poor gallbladder function

- Poor nutrient status (deficiencies of choline, taurine, magnesium, and others)

Therapies

Small intestinal bowel overgrowth therapies are designed to correct the balance of bacteria in the small intestines. Doctors begin treating SIBO by examining the cause of the underlying disease. Nutritional therapies and even antibiotics are also commonly required. Probiotics (good bacteria) are the mainstay of treatment, along with foods high in fiber and low in sugar.

LEAKY GUT SYNDROME

If you have dysbiosis, including SIBO, this commonly leads to what we first identified in Chapter 7 as *leaky gut syndrome*. Leaky gut syndrome occurs when there is damage to the lining of the bowel, which results in an increase of permeability. Intestinal permeability is a term that describes the control of material passing from inside the gastrointestinal tract through the cells lining the gut wall—and then into the remainder of the body.

The intestine normally exhibits some permeability, which allows nutrients to pass through the gut, while also maintaining a barrier function to keep potentially harmful substances from leaving the intestine and moving to the remainder of the body. Increased permeability allows toxins to re-enter the bloodstream and also, if you happen to be taking a prescribed dose of medication, to possibly get the medication a second time.

Symptoms and Signs

Symptoms and signs of a leaky gut may include:

☐ Abdominal pain   ☐ Anxiety

☐ Aches and pain in joints   ☐ Asthma

☐ Aggressive behavior   ☐ Bedwetting

- ☐ Bladder infections
- ☐ Bloating
- ☐ Chronic fatigue
- ☐ Chronic joint pain
- ☐ Confusion
- ☐ Constipation
- ☐ Cramps
- ☐ Diarrhea
- ☐ Exercise intolerance
- ☐ Fatigue
- ☐ Fever of unknown cause
- ☐ Flatulence
- ☐ Foggy thinking
- ☐ Food sensitivities
- ☐ Indigestion
- ☐ Inflammatory skin conditions
- ☐ Learning disorders
- ☐ Mood swings
- ☐ Muscle pains
- ☐ Nervousness
- ☐ PMS
- ☐ Recurring infections
- ☐ Shortness of breath
- ☐ Skin rash

Causes of Increased Intestinal Permeability

As we have already established in this book, there is no *single* cause for leaky gut syndrome. There are, however, several feasible reasons for its development. Some of the underlying causes of leaky gut include:

- Aging process
- Celiac disease
- Chronic alcoholism
- Diarrhea
- Food allergies
- Inflammatory bowel disease
- NSAIDs drugs
- Nutritional depletions
- Protozoal infections
- Small intestinal bacterial overgrowth (SIBO)
- Strenuous exercise
- Stress
- Toxic exposure

Conditions Associated with Leaky Gut Syndrome

Multiple diseases may emerge or be amplified due to a leaky gut, and they may extend beyond the gastrointestinal tract—including, of course, breast cancer. Many people have a GI tract that is *not* healthy. The good news (as we first discussed in Chapter 7) is that the 5R program for gut restoration is able to help almost all individuals to have a healthier gut—and that, in turn, produces a far healthier immune system.

THE 5R PROGRAM FOR GUT RESTORATION

The 5R program for gut restoration was developed by the Institute for Functional Medicine. It is a complete and comprehensive approach that not only improves symptoms but also helps heal with long-lasting results. The aim of the program is to: address dietary changes; balance gastrointestinal bacteria; create a balanced system of detoxification; normalize digestion and absorption; and to promote healing of the gut.

As we have already established, there are five key points that make up the 5R program and they are: Remove, Replace, Repopulate, Repair, and Rebalance. A comprehensive 5R program takes roughly about three to six months to complete. It is essential that you are amenable to implement the challenging dietary changes of this program—simply put, you cannot attain the maximum therapeutic benefit without the *dietary* portion.

Therefore, it is crucial to start the gut restoration program by eating a healthy diet. One study showed that your diet has the most powerful influence on gut microbial communities, more than anything else that can be done if you are basically healthy to begin with.

1. REMOVE

The first step in helping to achieve optimal GI health is to remove anything that has a negative impact on the gut. Finding a trigger may not be initially obvious and therefore may take some time. Triggers may include the following: food allergies, stress, pathogens, medications, and even supplements. Furthermore, inflammation in your body increases intestinal permeability.

2. REPLACE

Once the offending agents are removed, the next step is to replace digestive secretions that are low or lacking in your body. You may be deficient in several elements that are fundamental to digestion, such as stomach acid, bile, and digestive enzymes. Even common everyday things you may do, such as microwaving, can cause digestive enzyme depletion. You also may be lacking in certain nutrients.

3. REPOPULATE

Repopulation (or Re-inoculate) is to restore the balance of good bacteria in your gut, which is absolutely crucial to your overall health and having optimal immune function. This phase of the program involves using probiotic foods, fiber-rich foods, and commonly a supplement to help beneficial bacteria flourish.

PROBIOTICS

Begin by repopulating the gut with probiotics, which are good bacteria. They improve the intestinal microbial balance. In addition, reintroduction of good GI *microflora* leaves less space for pathogenic organisms to populate. Specifically, research has found strong associations between strains of *Bifidobacteria* and *Lactobacillus* as well as *Saccharomyces boulardii* and improvements in *both* intestinal cell barrier function and intestinal permeability.

PREBIOTICS

After one month on probiotics, you can then begin to take prebiotics (which are agents that support the growth and integrity of the already-taken probiotics. In other words, prebiotics are food for good bacteria since they help the growth of beneficial bacteria. They have been reported to improve the expression of tight junction proteins (helps cells form a barrier that stops molecules from getting through), thereby decreasing intestinal permeability.

You may need to take probiotics and prebiotics for the remainder of your life. The best way to permanently change the gut microbiota in your body is to keep that diet of yours *healthy*.

4. REPAIR

The gut lining can be severely damaged during times when the body is inflamed, under stress, and exposed to long-term allergens. This increases the intestinal permeability of the gut which allows antigenic macromolecules to cross the gut epithelium (gut tissue) leading to chronic systemic inflammation, which then decreases the gut bacteria leading to leaky gut syndrome. Repair of the GI tract lining is needed to ensure proper absorption of nutrients, as well as medications. A healthy gut lining also promotes an optimal immune system, which decreases your risk of developing many diseases (including breast cancer and a reoccurrence of this disorder).

THERAPIES

Repairing the GI lining requires several therapies. Begin by eating a diet rich in amino acids, vitamins, and minerals. Decreasing inflammation is key in repairing the gut lining. Fish oil, chamomile (*Matricaria chamomilla*), Meadowsweet

(*Filipendula ulmaria*), and Chinese skullcap (*Scutellaria baicalensis*) all decrease inflammation. Citrus flavanones can improve the microbiota composition by decreasing pathogenic bacterial and stimulating the growth of good bacteria. In addition, the consumption of citrus flavanones has been associated with a lower risk of degenerative diseases, such as cardiovascular diseases and cancer. Demulcents are herbs or foods that have a protective effect on the mucous membranes of the body. They contain a large number of mucilaginous materials that have a direct effect on the lining of the intestines to soothe them. Likewise, demulcents also reduce the sensitivity of the digestive system to gastric acids, relax spasm, decrease leaky gut, inflammation, and ulceration. Moreover, goldenseal (*Hydrastis canadensis*) stimulates the immune response and destroys germs since it contains berberine and Licorice root (*Glycyrrhiza giabra*), which contains flavonoids called saponin glycosides, resulting in a protective effect on the gut. Glutamine is an amino acid that stimulates intestinal mucosal growth and protects the gut from mucosal breakdown.

5. REBALANCE

Rebalance, the fifth "R" in the program, is where your way of life plays a crucial role. It is necessary to address the external stressors in your life that may increase your sympathetic drive in the nervous system and reduce the parasympathetic drive. The sympathetic section generally functions in actions requiring quick responses, fight or flight. The parasympathetic section functions with actions that do not require immediate reaction, associated with relaxation, digestion, and regeneration.

With practices like yoga, meditation, deep breathing, good sleep, and other mindfulness-based practices, you can help restore hormone balance that will protect your gut and, subsequently, your entire body. It would be pointless to go through the first 4 **R**s of the gut restoration program, only to then go back to old eating habits, lack of exercise, stress, and other things that contributed to GI dysfunction to begin with. Thus, the *fifth* R is just as important as the others for optimal GI health.

THE GI TRACT AND THE IMMUNE SYSTEM

The mucosal immune system of the GI tract both controls the GI microbiome and depends on it.

As you have seen, not only is the microbiome of the GI tract important for a properly functioning immune system, the breast tissue itself has its own microbiome that must also be healthy to decrease your risk of developing breast cancer and reoccurrence.

SUMMARY

This section explored the importance of normal GI microbiota, which is of rich diversity, as well as the significance of an intact GI barrier. Both are needed to maintain optimal gut health.

The key to understanding gut health is an awareness that the GI barrier consists of multiple epithelial functions as well as the mucosal immune system. The GI barrier not only protects you against potential dangers from the GI lumen, but also allows food and liquid uptake, beneficial crosstalk to the good bacteria, and immune tolerance against harmless antigens. An intact GI barrier maintains gut health. Whereas disturbance of GI barrier (leaky gut syndrome) is increasingly recognized as an early but important step in the pathogenesis of various illnesses, both directly related to the GI tract and other parts of the body as well.

The management of gut flora to enrich its protective and beneficial role represents a promising field of new therapeutic strategies focused on prevention and treatment of many disease processes along with enhancement of the immune system to help prevent breast cancer as well as a reoccurrence. Lastly, one of the principal regulators of circulating estrogens is the gut microbiome. Consequently, in order for the body to break down estrogen and excrete it from the body, the GI tract must be healthy.

INFLAMMATION: ITS EFFECT ON YOUR IMMUNE SYSTEM

Breast cancer is an inflammatory disease. Inflammation is a signal-mediated response to cellular insults by infectious agents, smoking, toxins, physical stresses, and even elevated cholesterol. As a crucial part of the immune system's response to injury and infection, inflammation signals the immune system to heal and repair damaged tissue. Consequently, healthy immune systems use inflammation to fix an unbalanced body. A small amount of inflammation heals, however too much inflammation is linked to many major diseases. Therefore, inflammation has a major impact on the immune system. When you run a temperature after catching a cold or have bronchitis, when you have a cough or have other symptoms, they are related to the body's inflammatory process setting up a healing response. It also assists in building long-term adaptive immunity towards some microbes.

The body sets up an inflammatory response to try and defend itself against an infection, such as a virus, bacteria, parasite, or fungus, to set up a detoxification mechanism, to heal itself, and to kill cancer cells.

WHAT CAUSES INFLAMMATION IN THE BODY?

Before the body sets up an inflammatory response, the immune system must recognize a threat to the body from one or more of the following categories that are discussed at length in Dr. Nancy Appleton's book entitled: *Stopping Inflammation: Relieving the Cause of Degenerative Diseases* including infection, surgery, physical agent (such as ultraviolet or other forms of radiation), vaccinations, chemicals, disease process, smoking, free radical production, obesity, chronic fatigue, allergies, and AGEs (advanced glycation end products, a source of inflammation from the diet such as includes sugar-rich foods and the consistent consumption of *processed* foods). One of the main causes of inflammation, as you have just seen, is an unhealthy gut.

WHAT HAPPENS TO THE BODY IN AN INFLAMMATORY REACTION?

The primary goal of the inflammatory response is to detect and eliminate factors that interfere with homeostasis. The following are some of the inflammatory mediators produced by the body: chemokines, cytokines, eosinophils, free radical production, insulin, interleukins, leukotrienes, mast cells, prostaglandins, and serotonin.

Cytokines play a large role in breast cancer related to inflammation. Several cytokines regulate the inflammatory tumor microenvironment. Interleukin (IL)-1, IL-6, IL-11, and transforming growth factor-β (TGF-β) stimulate cancer cell proliferation and invasion and cytokine receptor activation and intracellular signaling by NF-κB accelerate tumor progression. TGF-β is the most extensively studied cytokine in breast cancer. TGF-β belongs to the TGF-β superfamily and is a major regulator of many processes, including proliferation, differentiation, migration, immunity, and apoptosis. TGF-β has two actions in tumor progression. As a tumor suppressor, it has antiproliferative effects in the early stages of tumorigenesis, but tumor cells in later stages evade this effect and progress in response to this cytokine.

FREE RADICALS

Immune cells produce free radicals while fighting off antigens that are invading the body. A free radical is a molecule that contains an unpaired electron which is in search of another electron to stabilize the molecule. Free radicals include reactive oxygen and nitrogen species, which are key players in the initiation and progression of tumor cells and enhance their metastatic potential.

In fact, they are now considered a hallmark of cancer. However, both reactive oxygen and nitrogen species may contribute to improving the outcomes of radiotherapy in cancer patients.

DISEASES RELATED TO INFLAMMATION

Inflammation plays a central role in healing, but chronic inflammation raises the risk of certain diseases including cancer.

Tumor Development

Inflammatory responses play decisive roles at different stages of tumor development, including initiation, promotion, malignant conversion, invasion, and metastasis. Inflammation also affects immune surveillance and responses to therapy. Immune cells that infiltrate tumors engage in an extensive and dynamic crosstalk with cancer cells.

Epigenetic disorders—caused by modifications of gene expression in organisms—such as point mutations in cellular tumor suppressor genes, DNA methylation, and post-translational modifications are needed to transform normal cells into cancer cells. These events result in alterations in crucial pathways that when altered trigger an inflammatory response which can lead to the development of cancer.

Many inflammatory signaling pathways are activated in several types of cancer, linking chronic inflammation to the tumorigenesis process. Immune cells that infiltrate tumors engage in extensive crosstalk with cancer cells. A range of inflammation mediators, including cytokines, chemokines, free radicals, prostaglandins, growth and transcription factors, microRNAs, and enzymes as, cyclooxygenase and matrix metalloproteinase, collectively act to create a favorable microenvironment for the development of tumors.

COMMON TESTS FOR INFLAMMATION

There are now several blood tests that your healthcare provider can order that will help determine if your body is inflamed. Such tests should be performed regularly as a preventative action and to monitor your inflammatory standing. They include: CRP and hsCRP, IL-6, TNF-alpha, cytokine profile test, interleukin-2 blood test, leukotriene test, sed rate, histamine test, eosinophil test, and GlycA test. GlycA is a newer blood marker that tracks systemic inflammation and subclinical vascular inflammation.

TREATMENTS

Research is beginning to show evidence that inflammation could be a factor in a wide variety of diseases and illnesses. Fortunately, there are now conventional and Personalized Medicine remedies that present scientific promise.

CONVENTIONAL MEDICINE THERAPIES

Conventional therapies are centered on non-steroidal anti-inflammatory drugs (NSAIDs) that are both prescriptions and non-prescriptions, steroids, and second tier medications that are immune-suppressants and hydroxychloroquine.

PERSONALIZED MEDICINE THERAPIES

You don't have to rely solely on prescription and non-prescription drugs to decrease inflammation. Improving your lifestyle can balance inflammation in the body as well. It's possible to enhance your immunity the healthy way, by improving your diet and taking certain vitamins and herbal preparation.

- **Diet.** Proper nutrition and a balanced diet can be fundamental in preventing illness, from a common cold to cancer. Dietary patterns high in refined starches, sugar, and saturated and trans-fatty acids and poor in natural antioxidants and fiber from fruits, vegetables, and whole grains, as well as poor in omega-3-fatty acids may cause an activation of the innate immune system. Most likely this is due to excessive production of proinflammatory cytokines associated with a reduced production of anti-inflammatory cytokines. Higher intake of fruit and vegetables lead to both a reduction in pro-inflammatory mediators and an enhanced immune cell profile. Avoiding the use of sugar or the intake of sugary foods and beverages can help to decrease inflammation. (See page 257 for a longer discussion on sugary foods and their role in cancer initiation and progression.)

- **Herbal Therapies and Nutrients.** Various dietary components including long chain Omega-3 fatty acids, antioxidant vitamins, plant flavonoids, prebiotics and probiotics have the potential to modulate your predisposition to chronic inflammatory conditions. These components act through a variety of mechanisms including decreasing inflammatory mediator production through effects on cell signaling and gene expression (omega-3 fatty acids, vitamin E, plant flavonoids). In addition, it reduces the production of damaging oxidants (vitamin E and other antioxidants), and it promotes gut barrier function and anti-inflammatory responses (prebiotics and probiotics).

Curcumin has been shown to help in the prevention of carcinogenesis. It also acts as a prooxidant in cancer cells and is associated with inducing apoptosis. Curcumin quenches free radicals, induces antioxidant enzymes (catalase, superoxide dismutase, glutathione peroxidase), and upregulates antioxidative protein markers-Nrf2 and HO-1 that led to the suppression of cellular oxidative stress. In cancer cells, curcumin aggressively increases ROS that results in DNA damage and subsequently cancer cell death. It also sensitizes drug-resistant cancer cells and increases the anticancer effects of chemotherapeutic drugs. Thus, curcumin shows beneficial effects in prevention and treatment including responsiveness of cancer cells to chemotherapy.

LOW-DOSE NALTREXONE (LDN)

Naltrexone, a non-selective antagonist of opioid receptors, is mainly used as rehabilitation therapy for discharged opiate addicts to eliminate addiction to maintain a normal life and prevent or reduce relapses. In recent years, there have been some novel and significant findings on the off-label usage of naltrexone. It is hypothesized that lower than standard doses of naltrexone (low-dose naltrexone) inhibit cellular proliferation of T and B cells and block Toll-like receptor 4 (protein coding gene), resulting in an analgesic and anti-inflammatory effect. Low-dose naltrexone is a prescription compounded medication that very effectively reduces inflammation including all forms of cancer, particularly breast cancer.

SUMMARY

As you have seen, the inflammatory response can be provoked by physical, chemical, and biologic agents, including mechanical trauma, exposure to excessive amounts of sunlight, x-rays and radioactive materials, corrosive chemicals, and temperature extremes. Furthermore, they can be provoked by infectious agents, such as bacteria, viruses, and other pathogenic microorganisms. Although these infectious agents can produce inflammation, infection and inflammation are not synonymous.

Breast cancer is an inflammatory process as you have seen. Helping your body decrease inflammation using the nutrients described in this chapter, along with the nutrients discussed under modifiable risk factors for breast cancer, will help prevent breast cancer as well as decrease your risk of have metastasis and/or a reoccurrence. In addition, LDN is a compounded medication that all individuals should consider if they have had breast cancer as well as a wonderful tool to help prevent breast cancer by decreasing inflammation.

Remember, it is all about balance. A small amount of inflammation heals. Too much inflammation is linked to almost every major disease process from infections to breast cancer.

SLEEP: GET A GOOD NIGHT'S SLEEP

Since the time of Hippocrates, the relationship between sleep and immunity has been the subject of discussion. A good night's sleep is paramount for proper functioning of your immune system. Studies have shown that sleep loss can affect different parts of the immune system, which can lead to the development of a wide variety of diseases including breast cancer.

Trials have revealed that if a person slept four hours a night it reduced their natural killer cell activity by about 72 percent, which increased their risk of developing viral infections and cancer. Furthermore, when individuals had reduced sleep, they exhibited an increase in the formation of inflammatory cytokines which are important in the development of many disorders, including immune system dysfunction. Lastly, studies have also shown that not only do sleep-deprived people feel sleepy, but also other changes occur. Changes take place in their molecular, immune, and neural networks that play a role in the development of an exhaustive range of chronic health problems, such as obesity, diabetes, and cardiovascular disease.

One way to estimate your sleep-length need is to observe the length of time you sleep toward the end of a relaxing 2-week vacation, when you are not under time pressure and are sleeping freely (awakening spontaneously, without an alarm, and going to bed when you are tired). Keep caffeine intake to no more than 2 cups of regular coffee or tea a day. During the second week, record your bedtimes, wake-up times, and length of sleep. The average of the sleep times across the week is an estimate of your natural sleep-length need.

CIRCADIAN RHYTHM

The time frame in which you sleep is also significant. It is important to go to bed before 11:30 pm and not rise before 5 am otherwise the circadian rhythm in the body will change. Your circadian rhythm is a natural internal process that regulates your sleep-wake cycle.

It is also of utmost importance to examine the fact that sleep and the circadian system exert a strong regulatory influence on immune functions. Studies of the normal sleep–wake cycle showed that immune parameters, such as numbers of undifferentiated naive T cells and the production of pro-inflammatory cytokines, exhibit peaks during early nocturnal sleep. Whereas circulating numbers of cytotoxic natural killer cells, as well as anti-inflammatory cytokine activity cells peak during daytime wakefulness.

INSOMNIA

Insomnia is a common sleep disorder complaint in breast cancer patients and has been shown to have a host of psychological and medical correlations and consequences. It is defined as difficulties with falling asleep, falling asleep but then awakening later, obtaining a deep sleep, and staying asleep throughout the night. Another key factor of insomnia is poor-quality sleep that does not alleviate fatigue in that you may experience non-restorative sleep. Regardless of how much sleep you get, if you have insomnia, you seldom wake up feeling fresh and ready for the day.

Non-restorative sleep may be classified by how long the symptoms are present. Temporary insomnia or transient insomnia, which is usually due to stress, lasts for less than a week. Short term insomnia can last from one to three weeks. Chronic or long-term insomnia may last for three weeks or more. Insomnia can drain not just your energy level and mood but also your health, job performance, and quality of life.

Insomnia is on the rise worldwide. An estimated 50 million to 70 million adults in the U.S. have chronic sleep and wakefulness disorders. These numbers are similar in other industrialized countries in proportion to the size of the country. Insomnia is more common in women (25 percent) than in men (18 percent), and its prevalence increases with age, affecting approximately 50 percent of elder people. Estimates of the prevalence of insomnia in cancer populations range from 23 percent to 61 percent and are higher than that found in individuals without cancer.

Most of the studies on sleep problems in cancer have been conducted in women with breast cancer. Savard and his group studied insomnia prevalence in 300 non-metastatic breast cancer women and found that 19 percent met diagnostic criteria for an insomnia syndrome with 95 percent of the cases being chronic insomnia. They also found that in 33 percent of cases the onset of insomnia followed the breast cancer diagnosis, and that percentage of the patients reported that cancer either caused or aggravated their sleep problems.

Other studies revealed that women with breast cancer also experienced shorter sleep duration and higher rates of nighttime flashes (67 percent) compared to healthy women (37 percent). In addition, further trials reported that fatigue is one of the primary complaints in cancer patients. Also, Koopman looked at sleep disturbances in women with metastatic breast cancer. The results showed that 63 percent reported sleep disturbance.

Adequate sleep is foremost for your overall health, hormonal balance, and immune function. Optimal hours of sleep are between $6^1/_2$ to 8 hours of sleep per night. Less than this time frame is not healthy and sleeping more than 8 hours a night is also not beneficial. Most people who say they do not need a great deal of sleep are pushing themselves to sleep less, and as a consequence, struggle to stay awake and function during the daytime. Long-term they are at risk for developing obesity and several other types of chronic illnesses including breast cancer. Multiple factors contribute to insomnia among patients with breast cancer including endocrine therapies, hot flashes, pain and discomfort from local therapy, and fear of reoccurrence.

CONVENTIONAL THERAPIES

Since chronic insomnia can last for a long time and can seriously affect one's well-being and quality of life, many people turn to conventional medications to find relief. The following are traditional medications that have been used to treat insomnia. Traditionally insomnia is treated by classical hypnotics, such as benzodiazepines and Z drugs (this class includes zolpidem, zopiclone, zaleplon, and eszopiclone), which both act on the GABA -A receptor. Potentially, they may have many side effects, including cognitive impairment, tolerance, rebound insomnia upon discontinuation, increase in car accidents and falls, abuse, and drug dependence.

Newer medications for insomnia, such as melatonergic agonist drugs, agomelatine, prolonged-release melatonin, ramelteon, and tasimelteon are now being used more commonly.

Innovative drugs that have recently come on the market target the orexin/hypocretin system. They potentially have fewer side effects in terms of drug-drug interactions, interactions with alcohol, less memory impairment, and dependence potential compared to classical hypnotics.

In addition, there is some evidence for the use of quetiapine, trazodone, mirtazapine, amitriptyline, pregabalin, gabapentin, agomelatine, and olanzapine as treatments for insomnia. These drugs may improve sleep while successfully treating comorbid disorders, disorders existing simultaneously, with a different side effect profile than the older medications. Other modalities, such as non-drug therapies and cognitive behavioral therapies, yoga, and mind-body programs have also been traditionally recommended.

PERSONALIZED MEDICINE THERAPIES

Conventionally, medications and cognitive behavioral therapy have been used to treat primary or secondary insomnia without looking at the etiology of the disease process itself. The following review examines the causes of insomnia as part of the treatment of this common disorder along with other therapies.

Diet

The right diet is an important part of the journey in curing insomnia. In creating a diet for insomnia, you need to avoid foods that could make it worse and consume foods that could make it better. It is important to avoid processed foods with preservatives and avoid all foods with stimulant properties.

A study revealed that a Mediterranean-style diet was associated with adequate sleep duration, less insomnia symptoms, and the participants were less likely to have insomnia accompanied by short sleep. Likewise, a low intake of vegetables and fish and a higher intake of sugary foods and pasta were independently associated with poor sleep quality in another trial.

Poor sleep quality was also associated with high carbohydrate intake in free-living Japanese middle-aged female workers. Reactive hypoglycemia (sugar crash within four hours of eating a high carbohydrate meal) has been shown to be an etiology of insomnia. Eat more frequent healthy meals. Complex carbohydrates—such as lentils, lima beans, and peas—have been shown to help you fall asleep, since they protect your blood sugar from highs and lows.

If you commonly consume foods that you have an allergic response to, you may experience insomnia due to an elevation of epinephrine and norepinephrine that occurs when you eat these types of foods. Allergy testing may be helpful since many allergies are sensitivities (IgG responses) and not true food allergies (IgE responses). The severity of symptoms ranges from mild to life-threatening.

Likewise, foods that contain stimulant properties cause the body to work harder to carry out the digestive process and removal of toxins from the body. These include aspartame, caffeine, excessive salt intake and sugar.

Exercise

Exercise is important for your body and mind, and it can also aid in getting a good night's sleep. Nevertheless, you need to be mindful of the timing. For some, exercising too late in the day can interfere with how well they rest at night.

A study revealed that exercise was beneficial to decrease sleep complaints. In fact, exercise provided similar results when compared with hypnotics, a sleep-inducing drug. Another study examined workers, particularly sedentary older workers, having sleep problems reported less high-intensity leisure-time physical activity. This data suggests that a vicious circle may indeed prevail between poor sleep and reduced leisure-time physical activity.

Exercise can be invigorating and may keep you awake. Change your exercise routine to the morning and see if this is helpful. In addition, higher body temperatures also interfere with sleep. This is another reason to exercise at least 4 hours prior to bedtime.

Electronics

Cell phones, tablets, computers and other electronic devices have become such an enormous part of everyday life that it is often hard to put them down producing poor sleep patterns. Your phone, TV, or computer may be the reason you're suffering from sleeplessness.

There's now little reservation among scientists that a relationship exists between screen exposure at night and sleep quality. The results of a study show ed that computer usage for playing/surfing/reading was positively associated with insomnia, and negatively associated with being most active and alert during the morning. Likewise, mobile phone usage for playing/surfing/texting was positively associated with insomnia and chronotype (one's propensity to sleep at a specific time in a 24-hour period) and negatively associated with being a morning person.

The blue light released by screens on cell phones, computers, tablets, and televisions decreases the production of melatonin, the hormone that regulates your sleep/wake cycle or circadian rhythm. Lowering melatonin levels makes it harder to fall and stay asleep.

Hormones

Insomnia can also be related to a hormone imbalance. A hormone disparity can result in sleep problems, and a lack of sleep can cause further hormonal imbalances. The following are hormone imbalances that may cause your sleeplessness are loss of estrogen, progesterone, and DHEA. If you have had hormonally related breast cancer you may not be a candidate for this therapy. In addition, as you have seen, melatonin regulates sleep, in addition, this hormone has many other functions as discussed earlier in this text including treatment of breast cancer. Lastly, insulin is a vital hormone that is naturally manufactured by the body and directs cells in the body to remove glucose from the blood and use it for energy. Scientists have discovered that insulin resistance (a condition in which cells fail to normally respond to insulin) is closely linked to loss of sleep. Insulin levels tend to also rise if you do not have good sleep hygiene. A study revealed that sleep restriction (5 hours a night) for one week significantly reduced insulin sensitivity which is a risk factor for the development of diabetes and breast cancer.

Neurotransmitters

Neurotransmitters are chemical messengers in the body. Their function is to send signals from nerve cells to target cells. These target cells include muscles, glands, or other nerves. The brain calls for neurotransmitters to regulate many essential functions, one being sleep cycles. The neurotransmitters connected with driving wakefulness and sleep include histamine, dopamine, norepinephrine, serotonin, glutamate, and acetylcholine. Ask your Personalized Medicine practitioner for a neurotransmitter test if you have insomnia. It is a 24-hour urine study.

Nutrients

In addition to medications and lifestyle changes, there are several nutrients and vitamins that may be therapeutic for insomnia and provide quality sleep. Studies indicate that some vitamins may improve your sleep. My personal favorite is magnesium in the form of glycinate or threonate. Magnesium taken one hour before bedtime may be helpful since one of the symptoms of low magnesium is insomnia. Magnesium increases blood melatonin levels, which helps to improve your quality of sleep. Magnesium has also been shown to be helpful for restless leg syndrome which is one of the causes of insomnia. Dose: 400 to 600 mg one hour before bedtime.

Herbal Therapies

Herbs have been used in the treatment of insomnia for more than 2000 years. According to scientific research, insomnia has been effectively treated by herbal formulas. Herbs recognized as effective sleep remedies include valerian (*Valeriana officinalis*), hops (*Humulus lupulus*), and lemon balm (*Melissa officinalis*).

Other Therapies

Cognitive behavioral therapies, yoga, and mind-body programs have also been shown to be beneficial. It is also important for patients and healthcare providers to be educated regarding the emerging data for cannabis-based therapy.

SUMMARY

Women with breast cancer are prone to insomnia for various reasons including a possible disruption of sleep due to increased frequency and severity of hot flashes associated with the breast cancer treatment, and possible increased depression, anxiety and fatigue levels following the breast cancer diagnosis. In summary, chronic sleep deprivation can be seen as an unspecified state of chronic stress, which negatively impacts immune functions and your health in general. The adverse effects of long-term sleep deprivation comprise an enhanced risk for various diseases as a result of a persistent inflammation on the one hand, as well as immunodeficiency characterized by an enhanced susceptibility to infections and a reduced immune response to, to an increased risk of developing breast cancer. Getting enough sleep is crucial to your overall health in many ways; from positively affecting cortisol levels in your body to dramatically enhancing your immune system as well helping you maintain a healthy insulin level.

SMOKING: HOW IT AFFECTS THE IMMUNE SYSTEM

Cigarette smoking is considered the most preventable cause of death in developed nations as well as a modifiable risk factor for breast cancer.

SYSTEMS AFFECTED BY CIGARETTE SMOKE

Smoking tobacco has various effects on your body systems. It affects the respiratory system, the circulatory system, the reproductive system, the skin, and the eyes, and it increases the risk of many different cancers such as breast cancer. Furthermore, cigarette smoke causes diverse changes in immunity that lead to heightened constitutive inflammation, skewing of adaptive T cell-mediated immunity, impaired responses to pathogens, and suppressed anti-tumor immune cell functions.

Although most of smoking-induced changes are reversible after quitting, some inflammatory mediators like CRP (c-reactive protein) are still significantly elevated in ex-smokers up to 10 to 20 years after quitting. This suggests a low-grade inflammatory response persisting in former smokers long-term. In addition, many immunological changes in smokers are not completely reversible after they quit smoking. In addition, cigarette smoking has a negative effect on your health due to what is in tobacco smoke including arsenic. Preliminary evidence suggests a potential relationship between levels of arsenic exposure and breast cancer risk.

TREATMENTS TO HELP YOU BREAK THE HABIT

Several treatments are available to help you quit smoking by getting you past your craving for nicotine. These include both conventional therapies, including behavioral support, and Personalized Medicine therapies.

Conventional Therapies

Since the development of nicotine replacement therapy (NRT) in 1978, treatment options have continued to evolve and expand to aid individuals in smoking cessation. Despite this, currently available treatments remain insufficient, with less than 25 percent of smokers remaining abstinent one year after treatment. The two main approaches to assist cessation are pharmacotherapy and behavioral support.

Personalized Medicine Therapies

Personalized Medicine therapies have also been shown to be beneficial for some patients, including novel therapies such as the nutrient n-acetyl cysteine (NAC) are displaying promising results. N-acetyl cysteine has antioxidant properties, both increasing glutathione and modulating glutamatergic, neurotropic, mitochondrial, and inflammatory pathways. Also, studies have found that people who smoke, and those who are exposed to secondhand smoke, have reduced amounts of vitamin C in their bodies. Smokers should take an additional 2,000 mg of vitamin C a day. Lastly, tai chi, acupuncture, yoga, hypnotherapy, and mindfulness meditation have also been shown to be helpful.

SUMMARY

If you smoke: find a way to quit! When you begin, it appears as if it is a long road, however after a few weeks it starts to feel like a hazy memory. It can seem daunting and unbearable at times, but using the suggestions in this chapter, you can get through it. If you give up your smoking habit while you are healthy, your body can heal from most, or all, of the damage done by smoking. The rewards and benefits are worth it. If you have already been diagnosed with breast cancer, it is paramount that you quit smoking to decrease your risk of a reoccurrence of the disease.

STRESS: MANAGE YOUR STRESS

We all deal with stress at some point in our lives. You experience stress when your body reacts to pressure from certain situations. It can be your job, a family issue, illness, or money troubles. Your immune system is inherently related to your stress levels. Stress is an all-encompassing concept that comprises both challenging circumstances that are stressful along with both the psychological and physical response to stress. One of the major systems in the body that reacts to demanding circumstances is the immune system. In fact, numerous facets of the immune system are associated with stress. In addition, excessive stress is a modifiable risk factor for breast cancer development. Moreover, breast cancer diagnosis, surgery, adjuvant therapies and survivorship can all be extremely stressful. A small amount of stress keeps you on your toes, a large amount of stress causes distress to the body.

HOW DOES STRESS INFLUENCE IMMUNITY?

Immune cells have receptors for neurotransmitters and hormones, such as norepinephrine, epinephrine, and cortisol, your stress hormone. They mobilize and traffic immune cells that prepare the body to mount an immune response, if needed. Recent trials have shown that immunological cells (for example, lymphocytes) change their responsiveness to signaling from these neurotransmitters and hormones during stress. Likewise, immunological responses expend energy and over time deplete the body of some of its energy stores. Consequently, chronic stress produces negative systemic changes in the immune system and the remainder of the body. Furthermore, the cumulative effect of daily stressors promotes elevations in inflammatory markers.

SUMMARY

Research concerning the stress hormone, cortisol, has shown the large toll that both acute and chronic stress have on the immune system which increases your risk of getting breast cancer. In addition, studies concerning the effects of stress on inflammation have demonstrated that chronic stress can increase the likelihood of the development of many different disease processes, as well as exacerbating preexisting conditions such as breast cancer. Therefore, it is paramount that you have your cortisol levels evaluated. The optimal measure of cortisol for the purpose of evaluating the stress response is by way of salivary testing. Testing for cortisol levels will not be accurate if you have been on steroids within the last 30 days.

Furthermore, many individuals with abnormal cortisol levels also have a thyroid that is not functioning to its full potential (hypothyroidism). It is important to always work on fixing the adrenal glands before thyroid medication is instituted; otherwise, the symptoms of depleted or elevated cortisol levels may be made worse. See the chapter on hormones and the immune system for a more extensive discussion on your stress hormone cortisol as well as your thyroid hormones. For most women, breast cancer diagnosis, surgery, adjuvant therapies and survivorship can all be extremely stressful. One of the best stress reduction techniques that you can employ is prayer.

SUGAR—MINIMIZE YOUR SUGAR INTAKE

Cutting back on the amount of sugar in your diet can help you reduce the risk of developing most disorders, and as previously discussed is a modifiable risk factor for the development of breast cancer. Substituting high sugar foods with healthful choices can help you obtain all the essential vitamins and minerals needed by your body, minus the additional calories. It may also help with weight loss which also improves your immune system and decreases your risk of getting cancer as well as a reoccurrence.

SUGAR

Sugar comes in many forms, some of which are not as easily recognizable.

- Agave syrup or nectar
- Barley malt
- Beet sugar
- Brown sugar
- Cane sugar
- Cane syrup
- Confectioners' sugar
- Crystalline fructose
- Date sugar
- Evaporated sugarcane
- Fructose
- Fruit juice or concentrate
- Galactose
- Glucose
- Granulated sugar
- High fructose corn syrup
- Honey
- Invert sugar is a liquid sweetener made from table sugar and water
- Lactose
- Liquid cane sugar or syrup
- Maltose (malt sugar)
- Maple syrup
- Molasses
- Powdered sugar
- Raw sugar
- Rice syrup
- Sucrose
- Sugarcane syrup
- Table sugar
- Turbinado sugar
- Unrefined sugar
- White sugar

Reasons Why Sugar Can Harm Your Health

An excess of added sugar in your diet can result in many negative health effects. It also increases your risk of developing breast cancer.

SUGAR SUBSTITUTES

Trying to minimize the sugar and calories in your diet? You may resort to artificial sweeteners or other sugar substitutes if you cannot have sugar. These sugar substitutes are food additives, and they are equivalent to the taste of sugar however they have less food energy. Artificial sweeteners and other sugar substitutes are found in a range of foods and beverages advertised as "sugar-free" or "diet," including soft drinks and baked goods. What are all these sugar substitutes found in foods and what role do they play in your diet? Let's examine each of the sugar substitutes.

- **Aspartame.** Aspartame, a non-saccharide artificial sweetener, is 200 times sweeter than sugar. Once your body processes aspartame, a portion of it is broken down into methanol. Methanol is toxic in sizable amounts, yet smaller quantities may also be worrisome. Since 2014, aspartame has been identified as the predominant source of methanol in the American diet. Research has recognized a link between aspartame and a host of conditions and possible following side effects.

- **Sucralose.** Sucralose starts with a sugar molecule and has three of its components removed and replaced with chloride. It provides no calories because the body does not recognize it as a food. Sucralose does not raise blood sugar but is 2,000 times sweeter than sugar. As of the FDA's approval in 1998, studies have surfaced about sucralose's possible negative side effects. The risks of consuming large quantities of sucralose may include diabetes, cancer, weight gain, and gastric issues. In addition, it may increase the development of hypothyroidism, since chloride may replace iodine in the body when using a lot of sucralose. Iodine is needed for optimal thyroid function. It is also an antibacterial, anticancer, antiparasitic, antiviral, and mucolytic agent.

- **Honey.** Honey contains small amounts of vitamins and minerals and is 20 percent to 60 percent sweeter than sugar. The primary argument behind the negative effect of consuming too much honey is the excessive amount of fructose existing in honey. This high proportion of fructose in honey diminishes the ability of the small intestine to metabolize nutrients appropriately.

- **Saccharin.** Saccharin, one of the oldest artificial sweeteners, has been used for over 100 years. Limited research exists on the side effects of saccharin; however, a possible link may exist between consuming saccharin in substantial amounts and high blood sugar and alterations in gut bacteria.

- **Stevia.** Stevia is extracted from a leaf and has no known side effects. It does not raise glucose or insulin (the hormone that regulates blood sugar) levels in the body.

- **Sugar alcohols.** Sugar alcohols are naturally occurring sweet compounds found in fruits and vegetables. Supplements are made from the fiber of birch trees. Sugar alcohols include: xylitol, sorbitol, mannitol, and isomalt. They may decrease the incidence of dental cavities. They fight plaque buildup and neutralize plaque acids. Sugar alcohols also increase your feeling of fullness. They have 40 percent less calories than sugar and have a minimal effect on blood sugar and insulin levels. The body produces up to 15 grams of xylitol per day from other food sources. Sugar alcohols are incompletely absorbed in the intestine and may have a laxative effect, especially if used in large quantities.

Other artificial sweeteners that are currently permitted in the United States and other countries include acesulfame potassium, neotame, and advantame, They are all similar to aspartame, and luo han guo fruit extract. Refined sugars (for example, sucrose, fructose) were absent in the diet of most people until very recently in history.

SUMMARY

Long-term use of added sugar can be a problem for many people and can result in numerous medical conditions including breast cancer. Sugar upsets the balance of all the systems in the body, especially the immune system. Like many things in life, moderation is the key to health. It is all about balance. Sweet snacking is a frequent behavior at times of stress. Find another method of stress reduction. Remember: *Stressed* spelled backwards is *desserts*!

THYROID HORMONE AND THE IMMUNE SYSTEM

As you have just seen in the chapter on hormones, thyroid hormones regulate most everything that goes on in the body, which also includes the immune system. In fact, thyroid hormones have an extensive effect on the immune system. Growing evidence compiled over recent decades has revealed a two-way crosstalk between thyroid hormones and the immune system. This interplay has been demonstrated for several pathophysiological conditions of thyroid functioning and innate and adaptive immunity. The immune effects of thyroid hormones, T3 and T4, on the body occur in the innate immune cell subsets: neutrophils, natural killer (NK) cells, macrophages, and dendritic cells. Both hypothyroidism (low thyroid hormone production) and hyperthyroidism (excess thyroid hormone production) have been linked in the medical literature to the development of breast cancer.

In addition, environmental toxins disrupt the endocrine system including breast and thyroid balance and can influence pathological processes in both organs related to immune function.

SUMMARY

As you have seen, circulating thyroid hormone levels have a profound effect on neutrophil, macrophage, and dendritic cell function. This phenomenon suggests that thyroid hormone metabolism plays an important role in the host defense against infection through the modulation of innate immune cell function. As you have seen previously, evidence exists that there is an association between some viruses and the development of breast cancer.

One interesting fact discussed in the medical literature suggests that if you are a cancer survivor, you have an increased risk of having thyroid cancer. The reverse is also true, a study demonstrated an increased risk of developing breast cancer as a secondary malignancy following thyroid cancer. Consequently, have your healthcare provider evaluate your thyroid on a regular basis for malignancy and also test your thyroid function every 6-12 months.

WATER: STAY HYDRATED

The next key to having a healthy immune system is to drink enough water. Water regulates every function in the body. Without adequate hydration, the body manages less effectively in so many ways. Staying hydrated, not only allows your body to obtain electrolytes and helps your bodily functions to work at optimum levels, but also helps your system naturally remove toxins and other microbes that may result in a number of medical conditions.

Water enables the kidneys to remove toxins; if you don't drink enough water, toxins will accumulate, compromising your immune system. Being hydrated assures that your blood will transfer oxygen to the cells in your body and it allows your cells to take in nutrients. Water aids in the production of lymph, which the body utilizes to circulate white blood cells and nutrients.

Nutrition is a key element in maintaining a strong immune system and being hydrated assists in carrying out the digestion of food. In fact, a medical study revealed that low water and liquids intake was a risk factor for the development of breast cancer.

There is no substitute for water. The average woman's body is 50 to 60 percent water. Drinking more water also helps promote weight loss since it makes you feel full, decreases fluid retention, and aids in burning stored fat. One of my favorite reasons to drink more water is that it helps flush toxins out of your system. Furthermore, intaking additional water helps to hydrate your skin to help in avoiding wrinkling and encouraging the smoothness and softness of the skin. Lastly, having adequate hydration energizes you and is a great therapy for fatigue. Being well hydrated also helps your immune system function optimally.

GETTING WATER FROM YOUR FOODS

By the process of metabolism, you are able to obtain some of the water that is essential through the foods you eat, such as fruits and vegetables. Apart from generally getting about 20 percent of your water each day from food, you also obtain nutrients as well.

If you think that drinking water is boring, then add an orange, lemon, lime, or other fruit to enhance the flavor. However, you can obtain some of the water you need by eating foods with a high-water content, such as apples, cherry tomatoes, carrots, and cantaloupe. If you are traveling, minimize your intake of caffeine, sugar, and alcohol in order to stay hydrated.

SUMMARY

Staying well hydrated helps to enhance your immune system. As outlined in this chapter, being adequately hydrated promotes better health, reduces fatigue, aids in digestion, oxygenates the blood, flushes toxins out, as well as having a therapeutic effect for many chronic disorders. It allows your body to better defend itself against microbes and to recover more quickly. For overall well-being, it is important to appropriately hydrate.

In addition, one medical trial revealed that women with breast cancer consumed 20.2 percent less water and 14 percent fewer total fluids than controls. The study concluded that low fluid intake, particularly of water, may be a risk factor for the development of breast cancer. More research needs to be done to verify this result. In the meantime, drinking more water is suggested since it helps your body detoxify.

HERBAL AND NUTRITIONAL THERAPIES FOR IMMUNE BUILDING

Natural remedies made from herbs help us take control of our day-to-day well-being and boost the immune system. Herbal therapies include echinacea, glycyrrhizin, elderberry, astragalus, ginseng, oregano, and garlic. Olive leaf extract and cordyceps are also beneficial. Some of these nutrients can be taken long-term and some are for short-term use only when you are near someone who is ill.

Nutritional therapies, such as zinc, selenium, vitamin D, vitamin A, chromium, and manganese, have been shown to be crucial for the growth and function of immune cells. In addition, other nutritional remedies are available to build the immune system, such as transfer factor, beta glucans, glutathione, alpha-lipoic acid, modified citrus pectin, colostrum and sulforaphane. (See page 277 for more information on sulforaphane.) Amino acids, such as carnosine, carnitine, arginine, and glutamine, have also been shown to be effective.

Discuss with your healthcare provider the role of each of these herbs and nutrients in your overall health and together decide on the right ones that would be perfect for building your immune system as well as maintaining a healthy one to prevent breast cancer and a reoccurrence.

CONCLUSION

This chapter of the book assessed how your immune system works. It also examined 10 key components to improve your immune system.

Alcohol in moderation is vital for everyone and abstinence if you have a strong family history of breast cancer is paramount. Exercising, whether you like it or not, is key for your overall health and prevention of all diseases including cancer. A healthy gut really does equal a healthy immune system. In addition, decreasing inflammation will help prevent all major diseases from heart disease to memory loss, to breast cancer. Lowering inflammation also builds your immune system. Good sleep hygiene, and stress management are also of utmost importance for an immune system that works perfectly. Studies over more than half a century have shown that smoking increases your risk of developing cancer, not just lung cancer, but also breast cancer. Furthermore, it is now known that smoking cessation also improves your immune system. In addition, staying hydrated and minimizing your intake of sugar will also improve your overall health and your immune system. Lastly, having perfect thyroid function minimizes your risk of developing this disease process along with a reoccurrence.

Your body's immune system plays a major role in whether you develop breast cancer, whether your cancer spreads, and if it recurs. This is an area of study that is not commonly explored by traditional medicine but is one that you, along with your healthcare provider, can significantly improve.

9

Looking Forward

Researchers are working to advance current options for preventing breast cancer, early detection of breast cancer, and breast cancer treatments. As treatments for breast cancer are becoming more individualized, research studies are searching for methods to personalize the breast cancer screening and to find procedures that would be appropriate for each woman's level of risk in order to reduce the danger of over diagnosis which may lead to unnecessary treatments.

The latest findings have shown that breast cancer is influenced by the gut microbiome. It appears to influence the risk, the response to treatment, the proliferation, and reoccurrence of breast cancer. This chapter presents an understanding of the important role the gut microbiome plays in breast cancer and the nutrients currently being used to treat breast cancer. It also explores a new breast imaging technique along with the newest therapy in breast cancer prevention and treatment.

THE BREAST MICROBIOME AND BREAST CANCER

As you have read, the human gut microbiome plays an integral role in the physiology of the body with some microbes being beneficial and some microbes being known to be harmful to your health, including organisms linked to cancers and other diseases related to inflammation. Interestingly, host-microbiome interactions can promote effects in the gut and in organs further away, such as the breast. These effects are influenced by many microbe-derived factors, including metabolites (free estrogens, short chain fatty acids, secondary bile acids, and vitamins), immune and inflammatory modulators such as cytokines and toll-like receptors (TLRs), receptors that are the first line of defense against microbes.

Consequently, the community of microorganisms plays essential roles in health and disease, in both the intestine and outside the intestine. Dysbiosis (an imbalance between the types of bacteria) of the gut microbiota causes dysfunction in the intestine, which leads to inflammatory, immune, and infectious diseases. Dysbiosis is also associated with diseases beyond the intestine through microbial translocation or metabolisms. Bacterial translocation is a phenomenon in which live bacteria, or its products, cross the intestinal barrier which leads to leaky gut syndrome. (See page 238.) Accordingly, intestinal bacterial translocation may play a marked role in the process and development of breast cancer and other diseases. Thus, dysbiosis of gastrointestinal microbiota not only has consequences for local diseases, but also for the breast.

Moreover, studies suggest there is a distinct microbiome in healthy breast tissue compared to breast cancer tissue further implicating the role of the gut microbiome in cancer development. This alteration in gut microbiota is also associated with changes in estrogen metabolism, which strongly correlates with breast cancer development. Gut microbiota that express the enzyme β-glucuronidase may increase estrogen bioavailability. The breast distinct microbiome can be changed by tumors and diet.

Dr. I. Banerjee and his colleagues detected unique and common viral, bacterial, fungal and parasitic signatures for each of the breast cancer types finding distinct patterns for triple negative and triple positive breast cancer samples, while the ER+ and HER2+ samples shared similar microbial signatures. Moreover, Dr. Alice Tzeng noted that estrogen receptor (ER)-positive tumors consistently had lower amounts of seven bacterial categories compared to ER-negative tumors. In contrast, six bacterial categories showed associations with progesterone receptor (PR)-positive status.

In addition, human epidermal growth factor 2 (HER2)-positive tumors had significantly higher abundances of seven bacterial categories compared to HER2-negative tumors. Meanwhile, six of seven genera that were relatively decreased in ER-positive tumors were more abundant in triple-negative breast cancer (TNBC) tumors. Another study described that normal adjacent tissue from women with breast cancer (DCIS, invasive lobular and ductal carcinoma) compared to tissue from healthy controls had higher relative abundances of *Bacillus, Enterobacteriaceae,* and *Staphylococcus.*

These findings indicated that the bacteria or their components might influence the local immune microenvironment and that an unrecognized link between dysbiosis and breast cancer may occur. Consequently, the breast and intestinal microbiota are important factors in maintaining healthy breasts.

Furthermore, in examining aggressiveness and invasiveness in breast cancer, especially hormone receptor-positive breast cancer, it is central to examine the role of intestinal microorganisms in metastatic spread of breast cancer. Toll-like receptors are transmembrane receptors, an essential component of the innate immune system. (See page 218.) They recognize pathogen-associated molecular patterns which are products derived from pathogens of bacteria, fungi, and viruses. Emerging evidence suggests a strong link between TLRs and breast cancer. In fact, invasive ductal carcinoma showed a significant correlation between pathological features and TLR4 expression.

Consequently, the breast microbiota may influence breast cancer development and growth not only by regulating local estrogen levels, but also by shaping inflammatory responses and immune trafficking in the tumor microenvironment. Immune balance in the gut relies on constant crosstalk (process inside a cell when the same signal is shared between two pathways) between the microbiota and host immune cells. By influencing metabolism, inflammation, and immune responses, the microbiome can regulate cancer initiation and progression at both local and distant sites.

It is hypothesized that similar interactions could occur between the newly described breast microbiome and local immune responses to influence breast cancer pathogenesis (development). Just as important, the breast and associated microbiomes may regulate therapeutic response and serve as potential biomarkers for diagnosing and staging breast cancer in the very near future. In short, the breast and intestinal microbiota are important factors in maintaining healthy breasts. Dysbiosis of both the GI tract microbiome and the breast microbiome can lead to chronic inflammation, inflammation-mediated carcinogenesis processes, and immune invasion of the breast tissue.

NUTRIENTS AS ADJUNCT THERAPIES TO CONVENTIONAL MEDICINE FOR BREAST CANCER

Traditionally, treatments for cancer employ four methods—surgery, radiotherapy, chemotherapy, and immunotherapy alone or in combination. This section of the chapter will explore phytochemicals (nutrients) that are currently being used for breast cancer. Phytochemicals are unique bioactive organic compounds, which are mostly secondary metabolites (substance made when the body breaks down food, drugs, or chemicals) obtained from plant sources. These therapies have good scientific support to their efficacy. Furthermore, drug resistance is a major reason for examining natural therapies to be used in conjunction with traditional therapies.

■ COENZYME Q_{10}

Coenzyme Q_{10} (CoQ_{10}) is a fat-soluble nutrient that is made in nearly all of the body's tissues. It is sometimes called ubiquinone because it is ubiquitous—present everywhere. It is well-known for the part it plays in generating energy in cells by boosting mitochondrial function and is also a free radical scavenger that reduces oxidative damage.

Studies have also shown that it helps prevent breast cancer. Moreover, a study revealed that CoQ_{10} supplementation reduced some of the important markers of inflammation and matrix metalloproteinases (MMPs) in people with breast cancer. Matrix metalloproteinases (MMPs) are the main extracellular matrix enzymes in collagen breakdown and are a target for anticancer drugs. Another trial revealed that coenzyme Q_{10} is an antioxidant that can target the mechanisms of breast cancer tumor progression. In fact, this essential substance performs a range of important functions in the body.

Unfortunately, the body makes less CoQ_{10} as you get beyond fifty years of age. Because this nutrient is so vital to health, it is highly recommended that you take it in supplemental form after that age. If you have had breast cancer, studies have shown that it is a key nutrient to use in conjunction with conventional therapies for the treatment of breast cancer as well as to help prevent a reoccurrence.

Functions of CoQ$_{10}$ in Your Body

CoQ_{10} has many functions in the body. The most important is that it is a major part of the fueling source in your body called the Krebs cycle. It also functions as an antioxidant and studies have shown that it helps prevent breast cancer and is a wonderful treatment for peripheral neuropathy. (See page 42.)

Symptoms of CoQ$_{10}$ Deficiency

There are many symptoms of Q_{10} deficiency. The most common is generalized fatigue.

Causes of CoQ$_{10}$ Deficiency

The possible factors that cause lower levels of CoQ_{10} in your body are:

- Aging process
- Deficiency of taurine
- Deficiency of vitamins B_1, B_5, B_6, and B_{12}
- Excess exercise
- Folic acid deficiency
- Genetic mutations/genetic defects
- Hyperthyroidism (overproduction of thyroid hormones)
- Malabsorption due to celiac disease/sprue or steatorrhea (excessive fat in stools)

- Medications are a major cause of Q_{10} deficiency. Drugs from antibiotics to over-the-counter supplements used for weight loss can cause a deficiency of this nutrient. Speak to your healthcare provider or pharmacist to learn if any drugs you're taking might be causing CoQ_{10} loss.

Breast Cancer Benefits

Clinical trials suggest that CoQ_{10} may aid in treating breast cancer since it boosts the immune system, and it may possibly prevent the growth of cancer cells. In addition, it may prevent the proliferation of cancer cells.

Some chemotherapies deplete the body of this key antioxidant. Furthermore, Q_{10} has also been shown to help protect against cardiotoxicity or liver toxicity during chemotherapy. Therefore, coenzyme Q_{10} is suggested to be used during chemotherapy and other treatments for breast cancer and then to be continued lifelong.

Recommended Dosages

For the dosage specific to your disease process, see your healthcare provider. If you are over the age of fifty, 100 milligrams a day is a great starting dose. If you want to take a larger dose, increase the dosage slowly over a one-month period to help prevent side effects.

Some individuals may better absorb *ubiquinol*—the more active form of CoQ_{10}—than *ubiquinone.* When young, the body can readily convert ubiquinone to ubiquinol. With age, the body may be less able to produce the active form.

Side Effects and Contraindications

Do not use CoQ_{10} if you are pregnant or breastfeeding. If you take a blood-thinning medication, consult your doctor before using. Speak to your healthcare provider or pharmacist to learn if any drugs you're taking might make it unwise to use CoQ_{10}.

The following side effects can occur from taking CoQ_{10} supplementation. However, they are usually less severe if you take the supplement after meals:

- Abdominal discomfort

- Appetite loss

- Diarrhea (when doses are greater than 100 milligrams)

- Heartburn

- Increase in liver enzymes (when doses are greater than 300 milligrams)

- Insomnia (when doses are greater than 100 milligrams)

- Irritability

- Palpitations

- Photophobia (extreme sensitivity to light)

As you can see, if you are over the age of 50, your body makes less coenzyme Q_{10} and you would benefit from starting on this important nutrient. Coenzyme Q_{10} has also been effectively used to help prevent and treat many disease processes including breast cancer. It is suggested to start on coenzyme Q_{10}, 300 mg to 400 mg a day if you have had breast cancer

■ CURCUMIN (TURMERIC)

Turmeric has been used in India for over four thousand years as both a spice and a medicinal. Recently, science has revealed that the source of turmeric's ability to protect health is its main active ingredient, curcumin. Because of curcumin, turmeric has a surprisingly wide range of beneficial properties.

Function of Curcumin

Curcumin has been shown to have anti-cancer activity, is an antioxidant, and is anti-inflammatory. (See pages 206–207.)

Recommended Dosage

Take 400 to 600 milligrams daily. Choose a formula that includes piperine, a com- pound found in black pepper, or bioperine, which works like piperine. Curcumin is poorly absorbed when taken on its own, and these additions boost absorption.

Side Effects and Contraindications

If you are pregnant or breastfeeding, do not take curcumin supplements. Also avoid this supplement if you have gallstones, since it stimulates the gallbladder to produce bile.

Curcumin can have blood-thinning effects. If you have a bleeding disorder or are taking a medication or supplement that may thin your blood, do not take this herb. If you are planning to have surgery, discontinue this herbal therapy two weeks before the procedure.

Curcumin can also interact with blood sugar-lowering and immunosuppressant medications, as well medications that decrease stomach acid. Speak to your healthcare provider or pharmacist to learn if any drugs you're taking might make it wise to avoid curcumin.

Although curcumin does not cause significant side effects, the following can occur: dizziness, diarrhea, nausea, and stomach upset.

Breast Cancer Benefits

Curcumin has been reported to have anticancer and chemoprevention effects on breast cancer. Curcumin exerts its anticancer effect through a complicated molecular signaling network, involving proliferation, estrogen receptor (ER), and human epidermal growth factor receptor 2 (HER2) pathways. Curcumin has several specific diversified functions in breast cancer.

- **Proliferation.** Curcumin has been shown to inhibit NF-κB expression—arranges cellular resistance to invading pathogens. Therefore, curcumin is believed to show its impact on cell growth and invasion of breast cancer through the downregulation of NF-κB signaling pathway. Moreover, the Akt/mTOR-dependent pathway is a leading signaling pathway in the proliferation of breast cancer cells. Curcumin was found to inhibit the phosphorylation of Akt, mTOR and their downstream proteins, resulting in cell cycle arrest. Furthermore, curcumin suppresses breast cancer proliferation partially due to other trophic signaling pathways. In addition, curcumin also partially inhibited breast cancer cell growth by downregulating the insulin-like growth factor 1 (IGF-1) axis.

- **Hormone Factors.** Hormone factors also contribute to the growth and increase in numbers of breast cancer cells. HER2 and estrogen are the typical targets belonging to this category. A study found that curcumin and its analogues could work against HER2. Another study revealed that curcumin acts as a phytoestrogen which decreases endogenous estrogen which also contributed to the suppression of breast cancer cell growth.

- **Apoptosis.** Curcumin is reported to induce breast cancer apoptosis (cell death) by regulating the expression of apoptosis related genes. Curcumin was also reported to regulate apoptosis-related proteins.

- **Cell Phase Arrest.** Curcumin may also affect human breast cancer cells through inducing cell cycle arrest. Furthermore, the higher the dose of curcumin the better the response. In explanation, curcumin induces cancer cell phase arrest through regulating spindle-related signaling pathways.

- **Modulation of MicroRNA.** Curcumin suppresses breast cancer carcinogenesis partially due to modulation of microRNA, DNA, histone, and mitochondria.

- **Immune and Metastasis Factors.** Curcumin suppresses the growth of breast cancer by mediating the immune system in several ways. Curcumin can prevent the loss of T cells and inhibit immune suppressive cytokines, including transforming growth factor beta (TGF-β) and interleukin 10 (IL-10) in carcinogenesis.

- **Inhibits Angiogenesis Factors.** Curcumin also suppresses the growth of breast cancer by affecting metastasis by inhibited angiogenesis factors, such as vascular endothelial growth factor (VEGF) and basic fibroblast growth factor (bFGF)—tissue repair and regeneration, in ER-negative breast cancer cells.

- **Invasion.** Curcumin inhibits invasion and affects metastasis factors through invasion.

- **Reactive Oxidative Stress.** Oxidative stress is known to alter signaling pathways by damaging DNA molecules leading to the progression of breast cancer. Curcumin displays strong antioxidant activity which plays a crucial role against oxidative stress.

- **Oncogene and Tumor Suppressor Genes.** In certain circumstances, oncogenes are activated and reprogram normal cells to cancer cells. Treatment of curcumin resulted in a high level of tumor suppressor genes. Tumor suppressor genes prevent normal cells from being designated into cancer cells.

- **Curcumin as a Chemosensitizer.** Curcumin can serve as a chemosensitizer and can make tumor cells more sensitive to chemotherapy drugs. Curcumin can chemo sensitize anticancer capability. A similar mechanism can be found in doxorubicin-resistant breast cancer cells. A study suggested that curcumin reduced the expression of HER2 in doxorubicin-resistant breast cancer cells by enhancing the doxorubicin cytotoxicity by decreasing redundancy HER2 in breast cancer cells. Moreover, paclitaxel, another significant chemotherapeutic agent used in the treatment of breast cancer, has demonstrated acquired resistance in breast cancer cell lines. Curcumin has shown promising results in decreasing this drug resistance Furthermore, curcumin was found to enhance the sensitivity of breast cancer cells to cisplatin.

GREEN TEA / EGCG

Green tea has been popular in eastern countries such as China, India, and Japan for much of recorded history, and more recently, it has become popular in the western world, as well. It is recognized for a wide range of medicinal benefits which can be attributed to the many organic compounds it contains.

The most significant of green tea's anticancer components is believed to be *epigallocatechin gallate,* or EGCG which accounts for 50 percent to 80 percent representing 200 to 300 mg/brewed cup of green tea. One of a group of plant phenols described as tannins, EGCG is a powerful antioxidant that minimizes oxidative damage in the cells, helps protect against cancer (including breast cancer), enhances cognition, and benefits the cardiovascular system.

Green tea and black tea both come from the plant *Camellia sinensis,* but are different because of the processing used after harvest. While black tea goes through a lengthy process that includes oxidation of the leaves to form complex flavor compounds, green tea is simply steamed and dried. Therefore, more of the active compounds found in the tea plant are preserved in green tea. Benefits can be gained both by drinking brewed green tea and by taking EGCG supplements.

Breast Cancer Benefits

Green tea has been studied for breast cancer chemo preventive and possibly chemotherapeutic effects due to its high content in polyphenolic compounds, including epigallocatechin-3-gallate (EGCG). It is widely studied for its cancer preventing properties and is known to possess antioxidant, anti-inflammatory, anti-proliferative, anti-angiogenic (stops tumors from growing), anti-metastatic, anti-genotoxic (reduce DNA damage), demethylation of DNA, apoptotic (cell death), and epigenetic effects (changes related to altered gene expression). It is generally agreed that much of the cancer chemopreventive effects of green tea are mediated by its polyphenols known as catechins. The major catechins in green tea are EGCG, (-)-epicatechin-3-gallate, (-)-epigallo-catechin, and (-)-epicatechin.

EGCG blocks cell cycle progression and regulates signaling pathways that affect cell proliferation (rapid increase in numbers) and differentiation. EGCG also induces apoptosis, negatively modulates different steps involved in metastasis, and targets angiogenesis (development of new blood vessels) by inhibiting VEGF transcription. Investigations have shown that oral administration of EGCG results in the reduction of tumor growth and in anti-metastatic and antiangiogenic (block the growth of blood vessels) effects.

EGCG works in many ways to help protect breast tissue. The following are mechanisms of action of EGCG in cancer management through regulating various cell signaling pathways that govern carcinogenesis and cancer progression. EGCG decreases oxidative stress and reactive oxygen species (unstable molecule containing oxygen, a buildup may cause damage to DNA and may cause cell death), inhibits angiogenesis, inhibits carcinogenesis formation, inhibits pro-inflammatory mediators, and enhances antioxidant enzymes.

It also activates tumor suppressor gene. Therefore, this natural agent could be useful either alone or in combination with conventional therapeutics for the prevention of tumor progression and/or treatment of breast cancer. Particularly, several studies identified the polyphenols as adjuvants to chemotherapeutic drugs in triple negative breast cancer. Consequently, EGCG has great potential in cancer prevention because of its safety, low cost, and bioavailability (ability to get into the body and do what it needs to do).

Recommended Dosage

To benefit from green tea, you can either drink brewed tea or take supplements of EGCG:

* Consume three to five cups of green tea a day. Choose your favorite from among the many great-tasting green teas now available. Do not take green tea directly with iron supplements since the tannins in the tea may bind to iron and decrease its absorption.

* Take 200 to 400 milligrams daily of EGCO, 200 milligrams of EGCG that is 98 percent polyphenols which is equal to three cups of green tea.

Side Effects and Contraindications

Do not drink green tea or use EGCG if you are taking a MAO inhibitor. Green tea can interact with a number of drugs, from lithium to acetaminophen to many antibiotics. Speak to your healthcare provider or pharmacist to learn if any drugs you're taking might make it unwise to drink large amounts of this tea or take a green tea supplement. Be aware, too, that green tea may reduce the body's ability to absorb folic acid and iron. If you have liver disease, do not drink green tea or take EGCG without contacting your healthcare provider.

Unless the product is marked "decaffeinated," green tea and EGCG contain caffeine. Although the amount of this substance is small compared with that found in coffee, it can cause insomnia and restlessness in some people. Decrease the amount of tea consumed if the caffeine seems to be causing a problem. Because of the caffeine, use with caution if you have high blood pressure, cardiac arrhythmia (irregular heartbeat), anxiety, psychiatric disorders, insomnia, or liver disease.

Some people have allergic reactions to green tea. If you experience any signs of allergy, seek medical help immediately. The most common symptoms are the following:

☐ Anxiety

☐ Closing of the throat

☐ Constipation or diarrhea

☐ Difficulty breathing

☐ Headache

☐ Hives   ☐ Nausea   ☐ Swelling of the lips,
                                                       tongue, or face
☐ Loss of appetite

▓ GENISTEIN

Genistein is a flavonoid with phytoestrogen properties. Genistein is known to
have mechanisms of action for cancer prevention and also works as an antioxidant. It is mostly found in soybeans (*Glycine max*). It has been shown that
certain foods are poor or lacking, for example, soy oil and soy sauce, while
other ones such as soybeans, soy nuts, soy powder, soy milk, and tofu contain
a variable amount of genistein. The most genistein-rich foods are those fermented (miso and natto). There is great variability regarding the isoflavone
content of different soy-based foods, not only between different brands, but
also between distinct lots of the same brand.

Functions of Genistein

The main positive effects of genistein refer to the protection against cancer,
especially breast cancer. It also helps prevent bone loss.

Breast Cancer Benefits

Although the mechanism of protection against cancer involves various aspects
of genistein metabolism, scientists attribute this effect to the similarity between
the structure of soy genistein and that of estrogen. This structural resemblance
allows genistein to displace estrogen from its receptors, consequently blocking
their hormonal activity.

Numerous molecular pathways are targeted by genistein, which leads
to its anti-proliferative, anti-inflammatory, anti-metastatic, apoptotic, and
cytotoxic effects; it causes cell cycle arrest, reduces cell viability, and improves
radiosensitivity. A greater explanation follows.

- Genistein regulates estrogen receptor alpha (ER alpha) expression in breast
  cancer cells. It may decrease estrogen receptor alpha by reducing cell proliferation and differentiation. There are differences in cancer differentiation.
  A tumor that closely resembles the structure of the tissue it started in is
  described as very differentiated. Thus, the closer the structure of the cancer cell is to that of a normal cell structure, the better it is differentiated. A
  tumor that resembles the original tissue to a lesser extent is termed poorly
  differentiated, or anaplastic.

- It may also upregulate Bax and downregulate Bcl-2, leading to apoptosis
  (proteins regulating programmed cell death).

- Genistein decreases the methylation status (a process involving the addition of methyl groups to DNA molecules) and induces the expression of various tumor suppressor genes.
- It reduces the expression of DNMT1—an enzyme responsible for DNA methylation, leading to epigenetic modifications.
- In addition, it also represses cyclin B1 (overexpression may lead to uncontrolled cell growth), cyclin D1 (regulates the cell cycle), and induces BRCA1—when functioning properly, it prevents cell growth and prevents cancerous alterations in cells.
- Moreover, this nutrient downregulates molecular signaling leading to its anti-carcinogenic effects.
- Genistein also modulates miRNA (small non-coding RNA molecules) levels resulting in cell death.

Recommended Dosage

Many anti-carcinogenic effects of genistein are seen in the range of 10-20mg/kg body weight a day.

Side Effects and Contraindications

Intake of genistein through diet or supplementation has been shown to be generally safe. More research needs to be done concerning genistein's antioxidant, anticancer, cytotoxic, and anti-inflammatory activities, and its ability to be a therapeutic agent for diabetes, lipid metabolism, depression, neurodegeneration, bone health, cardiovascular disease, as well as breast cancer.

QUERCETIN

Quercetin is a flavonoid—a plant pigment—that is found in a number of different fruits, vegetables, grains, and other plants, including apples, red onions, purple grapes (and red wine), tea, and berries. It is also present in ginkgo biloba, St. John's wort, and American elder. One of the most studied of all flavonoids, quercetin is known to be a powerful and highly versatile antioxidant that has a wide range of important biological functions.

Function of Quercetin in Your Body

Quercetin has many functions in the body since it is anti-inflammatory and an antioxidant. There are many studies that show that it decreases the release of histamine which reduces the allergic response. In addition, it helps lower blood sugar and is an anti-cancer agent.

Breast Cancer Benefits

Quercetin is widely illustrated to have inhibitory effects on cancer progression through several mechanisms, including cell cycle arrest, metastasis and angiogenesis inhibition, antioxidant replication and estrogen receptor modulation. In addition, as you have seen, studies have revealed the other critical properties of quercetin such as anti-inflammatory. The anti-inflammation functions also through inhibiting the release of cytokines, decreasing the production of COX and LOX (enzymes associated with inflammation), and maintaining the stability of mast cells (white blood cells that are part of the immune system).

Quercetin also has a positive effect on proliferation and apoptosis that are considered to enhance breast cancer treatment. Induction of apoptosis is the ultimate goal in cancer therapy. Quercetin also prevents metastasis by reducing VEGF (a protein that stimulates the forming of blood vessels) secretion and matrix metalloproteinase (MMP) (play a role in formation of new blood vessels, immunity, and inflation) levels. Furthermore, it exerts its metabolic effect on cancer, inhibiting key enzymes of glycolysis—glucose is broken down to produce energy—and glucose uptake. In addition, this important nutrient inhibits angiogenesis. Quercetin also targets mitochondria in cancer, reducing bioenergetics and triggering intrinsic apoptosis (cell death). Furthermore, the effect of quercetin on glucose metabolism and cellular energy production contributes to its effect on cell viability reduction, decrease in metastasis, and apoptosis induction in cancer cells.

In other words, this important antioxidant has many functions that decrease the risk of developing breast cancer as well as helping prevent a reoccurrence. The ability of quercetin to target such a variety of molecular pathways makes it an ideal lead for anti-cancer drug development.

Recommended Dosage

Take 300 to 1,000 milligrams three times a day. For best results, always take quercetin with bromelain and vitamin C.

Side Effects and Contraindications

If you have a bleeding disorder or are taking a medication or supplement that may thin your blood, do not take quercetin, as this supplement may enhance the drugs' effects. If you are planning to have surgery, discontinue this herbal therapy two weeks before the procedure. Be aware that quercetin can interact with other medications, as well. Speak to your healthcare provider or pharmacist to learn if any drugs you're taking might make it unwise to use this supplement.

Quercetin may inhibit thyroid function. If you have thyroid problems, do not take this supplement without speaking to your healthcare provider.

Quercetin is an iron chelator and therefore inhibits the body's absorption of iron. Therefore, do not take quercetin at the same time that you are taking an iron supplement or eating a food that is high in iron. Wait at least two hours before or after taking iron to take quercetin supplement.

SULFORAPHANE

Sulforaphane is a plant compound found in cruciferous vegetables, such as cabbage, cauliflower, kale, broccoli, and especially in broccoli sprouts. This compound is stored in the form of glucoraphanin, a metabolite.

Functions of Sulforaphane

Studies have shown that this nutrient has many activities including being a strong antioxidant, anti-tumor, anti-angiogenic, and anti-inflammatory agent. Recently, newer drug delivery systems have been designed to enhance its availability to be effective and to reduce its potential side effects.

Breast Cancer Benefits

Sulforaphane has recently surfaced as a particularly potent chemo preventive agent based on its ability to target multiple mechanisms within the cell to control carcinogenesis. Sulforaphane exerts its therapeutics action by a variety of mechanisms, such as by detoxifying carcinogens and oxidants through blockage of phase I metabolic enzymes and by arresting the cell cycle. It may increase the levels of carcinogen detoxifying enzymes, decrease carcinogen activating enzymes, stop the growth of cancer stem cells, increase caspase activity which plays a crucial role in inflammation and cell death. Sulforaphane may in addition increase autophagy. Autophagy is the natural, conserved degradation of the cell that removes unnecessary or dysfunctional components. Very interestingly, sulforaphane enhances the activity of several classes of anticancer drugs including paclitaxel, docetaxel, and gemcitabine through additive and synergistic effects.

Recommended Daily Dosage

Dosing will depend on the active component contained in the supplement. Most common dose is 10 to 30 mg twice a day.

Side Effects and Contraindications

No side effects have been reported.

Sulforaphane may interact with medications changed by the liver's cytochrome P450 (CYP) enzyme. Therefore, use with caution in patients taking medications that pass through the liver.

OTHER NATURAL THERAPIES

■ MUSHROOM EXTRACTS

Edible dietary and medicinal mushrooms have been known to be a source that has health benefits and have been traditionally used in Asia. Wong and colleagues in their review demonstrate that mushrooms can be used medicinally as an adjunct therapy for breast cancer. Researchers found that mushroom extracts decreased the size of the breast cancer cells and slowed down their growth. In particular, a study found that the chemicals in mushrooms slow the production of estrogen. There has been speculation that white button mushrooms improve our immune function to fight cancer.

The mushrooms which are better known to have indirect or direct activity on breast cancer include the following:

- Brazilian mushroom Agaricus blazei
- Button mushroom Agaricus bisporus
- Maitake mushroom or sheep's head mushroom Grifola frondosa
- Oyster mushroom Pleurotus ostreatus
- Reishi mushroom or Lingzhi Ganoderma lucidum
- Shiitake mushroom (Lentinula edodes)

In addition, anticancer mechanisms in human clinical trials have been reported for:

- Antrodia camphorate
- Cordyceps sinensis
- Lentinula edodes

▨ SODIUM BUTYRATE

Sodium butyrate is a short-chain fatty acid and the byproduct of carbohydrate metabolism in the gut. Maintaining optimal butyrate levels improves gastrointestinal health in animal models by supporting colonocyte function (cells lining the colon that maintain homeostasis), decreasing inflammation, maintaining the gut barrier, and promoting a healthy microbiome. Butyrate has also shown protective actions in intestinal diseases and colon cancer and breast cancer.

Several mechanisms are proposed to be involved in the regulation of cancer cell growth induced by sodium butyrate including the inhibition of DNA double strand break repair and the lowering of oxidative stress. Moreover, butyrate is important as food for cells lining the colon and also serves as a histone deacetylase inhibitor which can promote apoptosis (cell death) and ultrastructural changes, as well as enhance anti-tumor activity. The balance between apoptosis and proliferation determines the balance of cell growth.

Excitingly, sodium butyrate and other HDAC inhibitors (changes the way histones—proteins found in chromosomes—bind to DNA) have shown promising therapeutic outcomes against triple-negative breast cancer, especially if they are used in combination with other anticancer agents. It is suggested that your anti-aging/Personalized Medicine practitioner order a gut health test to determine if taking sodium butyrate would be beneficial for you.

SUMMARY

Fortunately, there are several natural therapies that can be used as adjunct treatments to conventional care for breast cancer that have been found in clinical trials to be effective. Chromium, coenzyme Q_{10}, sulforaphane, quercetin, genistein, and curcumin amongst them as well as mushroom extracts and sodium butyrate.

DIAGNOSTIC TOOLS

There are now new diagnostic tools that are available to help measure how fast the cancer cells are growing and dividing.

▨ PERFEQTION IMAGING: THE NEWEST IMAGING TECHNIQUE

A new imaging technique has been newly developed by Jennifer Simmons, M.D. It is called PerfeQTion Imaging. It is a cutting-edge technology to screen for breast cancer. The imaging uses sound waves to create a 3D reconstruction of the breast in minutes with 40 times the resolution of an MRI.

This revolutionary approach offers a safe, comfortable, fast, radiation-free, and efficient possible alternative to the current breast imaging methods. Since this is a new technique, further studies need to be done, but PerfeQTion offers a new modality to evaluate breast health that may in the future replace some of the older techniques.

A NEW THERAPY

While there are a number of new therapies now on the horizon, therapeutic plasma exchange (TPE), also known as plasma exchange therapy, is the one that is the most promising.

Therapeutic Plasma Exchange (TPE)

Therapeutic plasma exchange is a procedure where the plasma in your blood is removed and replaced with another fluid. This is somewhat like kidney dialysis. This therapy has been available for over 50 years and early on, it was used in hospital emergency departments to remove medications that were overdosed or accidentally ingested by patients before the drug naltrexone (Narcan) was introduced. TPE is currently being used for neurological disorders such as multiple sclerosis and blood disorders.

As previously discussed, bisphenol A (BPA) is related to the development of several forms of cancer including breast cancer. In fact, BPA increases ductal density and sensitivity to estrogens after BPA exposure, which is generally shown in human breast cancer development. Furthermore, large-scale epigenetic changes from fetal BPA exposure may lead to altered gene expression patterns, intraductal hyperplasia, and ductal carcinomas in situ (DCIS) in adults. In addition, BPA promotes carcinogenesis of breast cancer by affecting the environment surrounding mammary epithelial cells. BPA may also adversely influence various cell types within the gland, such as fibroblasts, adipocytes, and immune cells, thus changing soluble factor secretion, extracellular matrix components and organization, and the local immune context. These alterations can lead to chronic inflammation, modification of tissue homeostasis (tissue stability), and neoplastic transformation of epithelial cells of the breast.

BPAs can be measured in your urine. They are, however, not commonly requested by your healthcare provider since until very recently the medical science was not here to help remove them from your system. In the last couple of years, a new technique using therapeutic plasma replacement (TPE) was developed for the removal of toxins from the body such as BPA. TPE as a therapy that is common and a relatively safe treatment. It is a technique which is performed outside the body using a devise that separates and removes specific components of the blood. In this technique, your plasma is separated from whole blood and removed, while the cellular blood components are returned to you together with a replacement fluid such as albumin.

By the removal of harmful substances, such as BPA, and the replacement of deficient plasma components with the addition of nutrients, this technique constitutes an important new therapy for the possible prevention of breast cancer as well as decreasing the risk of a reoccurrence. Moreover, TPE with the addition of chelating agents such as DMSA, have been shown to remove heavy metals from the body, some of which are related to an increased risk of developing breast cancer like cadmium, copper, and lead.

CONCLUSION

As you have seen, the latest findings have shown that breast cancer is influenced by the gut microbiome. It influences the risk, the response to treatment, the proliferation, and possible reoccurrence of this disease. There are also several phytonutrients that have clinical evidence that they are an effective therapy for breast cancer. Overall, these phytonutrients are found to inhibit breast cancer cell proliferation, differentiation, invasion, metastasis, angiogenesis, and induce apoptotic cell death by targeting various molecular pathways. They also alter epigenetic mechanisms and enhance the chemosensitivity and radiosensitivity of cancer cells. Their use is something that should be considered as adjunct therapy to conventional treatments for breast cancer. Lastly, new imaging techniques and new cancer markers have been unmasked along with novel therapies in this ever-changing landscape of breast cancer prevention and treatment.

Conclusion

The incidence of breast cancer cases is expected to increase by more than 46 percent by the year 2040. As a woman, I understand how scary that statistic is; however, as a physician, I also know that there are things you can do *now* to avoid or greatly reduce your odds of getting breast cancer. My goal in writing this book has been to provide a comprehensive approach to the prevention of breast cancer, so that these numbers will not be a reality. And just as important, it is also my goal to significantly decrease the incidence of its reoccurrence.

If you have had breast cancer and have been through treatment, your biggest fear might be that it may come back. While there is no way to predict if your cancer will return, do not let fear control your life. As you have seen, research shows that making lifestyle changes that are modifiable can aid you in staying as healthy as possible and may reduce your risk of developing this disease again. Moreover, building your immune system will also go a long way in preventing a reoccurrence of breast cancer.

Part 1 of this book looked at what breast cancer is. It then examined the types of breast cancers found, the various ways breast cancer is diagnosed, and the conventional treatments used to combat it. This section also reviewed three major possible side effects of cancer therapies. This includes neuropathy (nerve damage caused by chemotherapy or other conditions, which often leads to weakness, numbness, and pain in your hands and feet), osteoporosis (bone loss), and a weakened immune system.

Part 2 first explored your unchangeable risk factors for breast cancer. These are the ones that you cannot change. However, the sooner you learn about some of these higher-risk factors, the sooner you will see how some of them may actually be reduced, such as the age when you may choose to have children.

From there, we covered your controllable risk factors. These are the ones that you have control over: the body's ability to break down estrogen; your sugar and alcohol intake; whether you are obese, and if you exercise; whether your cholesterol level is elevated; if you methylate properly; if you have an optimal level of vitamin D; how healthy your GI tract is; and if your body is inflamed. Moreover, a wide array of chronic inflammatory conditions predisposes susceptible cells to neoplastic transformation. Consequently, decreasing inflammation is something you should strive to do daily. In general, the longer the inflammation persists, the higher your risk of cancer.

Just as important, we have explored a chapter that assesses how your immune system works. Your body's immune system plays a major role in whether you develop breast cancer, whether your cancer spreads, and if it reoccurs. This is an area of study that is not commonly explored by traditional medicine. This section also looked at the future perspectives on the prevention, diagnosis, and treatment of breast cancer.

The interesting fact is that there is an interplay between your controllable risk factors and what methods you can employ to improve and optimize your immune system. Many of these elements are the same. For example, smoking increases your risk of developing breast cancer, and it also weakens your immune system. If you have a vigorous exercise program, it decreases your risk of acquiring breast cancer as well as aids in building and maintaining a robust immune system. If any part of your body's internal systems is inflamed, it increases your risk of developing this potentially devastating disease and compromises your immune system. Certainly, your hormones affect both your risk of developing breast cancer as well as how your immune system works.

Consequently, there are 16 key components of living and looking at your health that you can do to help prevent this potentially devastating disease, along with stopping it from occurring again.

TOP 16 THINGS YOU CAN DO TO HELP PREVENT BREAST CANCER AND A REOCCURRENCE

1. Reduce stress.

2. Decrease your intake of alcohol.

3. Lower your ingestion of sugar.

4. See a Personalized Medicine specialist to help balance your hormones.

5. Make sure you methylate effectively.

6. Reduce your risk of developing insulin resistance. (If you already have it, then work on effectively managing this disease process.)

7. Look at how your body breaks down estrogen and ensure that it is optimal.

8. Eat a Mediterranean diet.

9. Drink enough purified water.

10. Reduce your exposure to toxins.

11. Have good sleep hygiene.

12. Exercise three to four days a week.

13. Be an optimal weight.

14. Do not smoke.

15. Reduce inflammation in your body.

16. Have a healthy GI tract.

Fortunately, as you have seen, there are also many methods to help you decrease your risk of developing breast cancer and/or having it reoccur, if you have already had this disease. The fact is breast cancer is *preventable* in many people. The great news is that you have the power to incorporate most, or all, of these changeable risk factors into your life. You can also build up your immune system to decrease your risk of developing breast cancer, lower your risk of the cancer spreading, and reduce the chance of this disease from coming back. Happily, new therapies are being developed on a regular basis. The science is now here to personalize your health care, from prevention to treatment. All you have to do is take advantage of it.

Resources

In this book, I have tried to provide all the information you need to understand breast cancer, including how to hopefully prevent it, and—if you have already *had* this disease—how to potentially stop a recurrence. Although you can put together and follow this regimen on your own, it is often helpful to work with a Personalized Medicine specialist and/or compounding pharmacist who can customize your program to your own special needs. If you have had breast cancer, it is also extremely important to continue to work with your oncologist and to see them on a regular basis.

Whether you design your own regimen, rely on the guidance of a medical specialist, or the counsel of a pharmacist, you will benefit most if you use pharmaceutical-grade supplements, which meet the highest regulatory requirements.

The following lists will guide you to the resources that can help you realize your goals of cancer prevention; avoiding a recurrence; maximizing your immune system; and optimizing your health.

BREAST CANCER ORGANIZATIONS

The following organizations are designed to provide both information and support on all aspects of breast cancer. It is important to know that you are not alone. These organizations can help connect you with those who can answer your questions best.

American Cancer Society (ACS)
The American Cancer Society is a voluntary health organization whose aim is to fight cancer through research, advocacy, and patient support. Based on where a patient resides, they offer free transportation and lodging as well as a free 24-hour helpline.
Phone: 1-800-227-2345
Website: www.cancer.org

The National Breast Cancer Foundation (NBCF)
The National Breast Cancer Foundation is a US-based breast cancer organization that promotes breast cancer awareness and education, provides free screening services, and supports patients and survivors.
Phone: 1-972-248-9200
Website: www.nationalbreastcance.org

The American Breast Cancer Foundation

The American Breast Cancer Foundation is a charitable organization focused on breast cancer prevention. Based in Columbia, Maryland, the organization provides early detection, education, and screening services.
Phone: 1-844-219-2223
Website: www.abcf.org/

Susan G. Komen Breast Cancer Foundation

This is a non-profit organization that promotes education, advocates for access to screening and treatment, and provides a number of patient support services. This includes grants for medications, medical equipment, local transportation, and childcare.
Phone: 1-877-465-6636
Website: www.komen.org/

FINDING A COMPOUNDING PHARMACY

Compounding is the practice of creating personalized medications to fill the gaps left by mass-produced medicine. To meet the special needs of an individual, a compounding pharmacy can provide unique dosages, innovative delivery methods, and unusual flavorings, and can also eliminate allergens and unnecessary fillers. **Professional Compounding Centers of America** can help you find a PCCA-member pharmacy in your area.

Professional Compounding Centers of America
9901 South Wilcrest Drive
Houston, TX 77099
Phone: 1-800-331-2498
Website: www.pccarx.com

Alliance for Pharmacy Compounding
100 Daingerfield Road., Suite 100
Alexandria, VA 22314
Phone: 1-281-933-8400
Website: www.a4pc.org
        www.compounding.com

DIAGNOSTIC LABORATORY CONTACT INFORMATION

Medical testing now makes it possible to measure your amino acids, fatty acids, organic acids, vitamin levels, hormone levels, gastrointestinal function, genome, and much more. This means that your regimen can be personalized to meet your specific needs. The following laboratories can perform tests to evaluate many important aspects of your health. Before ordering any medical test(s), be sure to consult with your healthcare practitioner.

Access Medical Labs
5151 Corporate Way
Jupiter, FL 33458

Phone: 1-866-720-8386 x 120
Website: www.accessmedlab.com

Cyrex Laboratories
2602 South 24th Street
Phoenix, AZ 85034
Phone: 1-877-772-9739 (US)
   1-844-216-4763 (Canada)
Website: www.cyrexlabs.com

Doctor's Data
3755 Illinois Avenue
St. Charles, IL 60174
Phone:1-800-323-2784
Website: www.doctorsdata.com

Genova Diagnostics
63 Zillicoa Street
Asheville, NC 28801
Phone: 1-800-522-4762
   1-828-253-0621
Website: www.gdx.net

Microbiome Labs Research Center
1332 Waukegan Road
Glenview, IL 60025
Phone: 1-904-940-2208
Website: www.biomeFx.com

Vibrant America Labs
1021 Howard Avenue
San Carlos, CA 94070
Phone: 1-866-364-0963
Website: www.vibrant-america.com

ZRT Laboratory
8605 SW Creekside Place
Beaverton, OR 97008
Phone: 1-866-600-1636
   1-503-466-2445
Website: www.zrtlab.com

PHARMACEUTICAL-GRADE COMPANIES

You can find many good supplement brands at health food stores. Always make sure you buy pharmaceutical-grade nutrients. The following pharmaceutical-grade companies offer many top quality nutritional supplements. Contact them for full product lists, as well as for directions on how best to order their products.

Biotics Research Corporation
6801 Biotics Research Drive
Rosenberg, TX 77471
Phone: 1-800-231-5777
   1-281-344-0909
Website: www.bioticsresearch.com

Designs for Health, Inc.
980 South Street
Suffield, CT 06078
Phone:1-800-847-8302
   1-860-623-6314
Website: www.designsforhealth.com

Douglas Laboratories
112 Technology Drive
Pittsburgh, PA 15275
Phone: 1-800-245-4440
Website: www.douglaslabs.com

Metagenics
25 Enterprise
Aliso Viejo, CA 92656
Phone: 1-800-692-9400
   1-949-366-0818
Website: www.metagenics.com

Microbiome Labs
1332 Waukegan Road
Glenview, IL 60025
Phone: 1-904-940-2208
Website: microbiomelabs.com

Ortho Molecular Products
1991 Duncan Place
Woodstock, IL 60098
Phone:1-800-332-2351
Website:
    www.orthomolecularproducts.com

Vital Nutrients
45 Kenneth Dooley Drive
Middletown, CT 06457
Phone: 1-888-328-9992
    1-860-638-3675
Website: www.vitalnutrients.net

Xymogen
6900 Kingspointe Parkway
Orlando, FL 32819
Phone: 1-800-647-6100
Website: www.xymogen.com

References

The information and recommendations presented in this book are based on over a thousand scientific studies, academic papers, and books. If the references for all these sources were printed here, they would add considerable bulk to the book and make it more expensive, as well. For this reason, the publisher and I have decided to present a complete list of references, categorized by section and topic, on the publisher's website. This format has the added advantage of enabling us to make you aware of further important studies and papers as they become available. You can find the references under the listing of my book at www.squareonepublishers.com.

About the Author

Pamela Wartian Smith, MD, MPH, MS, spent her first twenty years of practice as an emergency room physician with the Detroit Medical Center and then spent the next twenty-eight years of her career as an Anti-Aging/Functional Medicine specialist. She is a diplomate of the board of the American Academy of Anti-Aging Physicians and an internationally known speaker and author on the subject of Anti-Aging/Precision Medicine. She holds a master's degree in public health as well as in metabolic and nutritional medicine. Dr. Smith is currently in private practice and the senior partner for the Center for Precision Medicine, with offices in Michigan and Florida. She is also the founder of the Fellowship in Anti-Aging, Regenerative, and Functional Medicine and the past co-director of the master's program in metabolic and nutritional medicine at the Morsani College of Medicine, University of South Florida.

Dr. Smith has been a featured guest on CNN, PBS, and a number of other television networks, in addition to hosting two radio shows. She can also be seen in the PBS series *The Embrace of Aging,* the online medical series *Awakening from Alzheimer's* and *Regain Your Brain,* and the PBS/CNN special *How to Maximize Your Immune System.* She is the author of eleven best-selling books, including *What You Must Know About Vitamins, Minerals, Herbs, and So Much More; What You Must Know About Women's Hormones;* and *Max Your Immunity.*

Index